PSYCHOLOGY OF LEARNING AND HUMAN DEVELOPMENT

PSYCHOLOGY OF LEARNING AND HUMAN DEVELOPMENT

As per New Syllabus of Tamil Nadu Teachers Education University

Babu Muthuja
M.A., M.A., M.Ed.
Educational Advisor,
Arcot Sri Mahalakshmi Matric Hr. Sec. School,
Villapakkam, Vellore Dist.-632521 T.N.

R. Usharani
M.A., M.Ed.
Principal, Arcot Sri Mahalakshmi Matric Hr. Sec. School,
Villapakkam, Vellore Dist.-632521 T.N.

Dr. Anamika
Lecturer, Deptt. of Education
Drona College of Management and Technical Education,
Dehradun

CENTRUM PRESS
NEW DELHI-110002 (INDIA)

CENTRUM PRESS
H.O.: 4360/4, Ansari Road, Daryaganj,
New Delhi-110 002 (India)
Ph.: 23278000, 23261597
B.O.: No. 1015, Ist Main Road, BSK IIIrd Stage
IIIrd Phase, IIIrd Block,
Bangalore - 560 085 (India)
Tel.: 080-41723429
Visit us at: www.centrumpress.com

Psychology of Learning and Human Development

First Edition, 2009

PRINTED IN INDIA

Printed at Balaji Offset, Delhi

Contents

Preface

Learning is often defined as a relatively permanent change in behavior as a result of experience. Learning is a process that depends on experience and leads to longterm changes in behavior potential. Behavior potential designates the possible behavior of an individual, not actual behavior. The main assumption behind all learning psychology is that the effects of the environment, conditioning, reinforcement, etc. provide psychologists with the best information from which to understand human behavior. As opposed to *short term* changes in behavior potential (caused e.g. by fatigue) learning implies *long term* changes. As opposed to long term changes caused by *aging and development*, learning implies changes related directly to *experience*.

Learning theories try to better understand how the learning process works. Major research traditions are behaviorism, Cognitivism (psychology) and self-regulated learning. Neurosciences have provided important insights into learning, too, even when using much simpler organisms than humans (aplysia).' Developmental psychology', also known as human development, is the scientific study of systematic psychological changes that occur in human beings over the course of the life span. Originally concerned with infants and children, the field has expanded to include adolescence and adult development, aging, and the entire life span. This field examines change across a broad range of topics including motor skills and other psycho-physiological processes; cognitive development involving areas such as problem solving, moral understanding, and conceptual understanding; language acquisition; social, personality, and emotional development; and self-concept and identity formation. Developmental psychology includes issues such as the extent to which development occurs through the gradual accumulation of knowledge versus stage-like development, or the extent to which children are born with innate mental structures versus learning through experience. Many researchers are interested in the interaction between personal characteristics, the individual's behavior, and environmental factors including social context, and their impact on development; others take a more narrowly focused approach.

Developmental psychology informs several applied fields, including: educational psychology, child psychopathology, and forensic developmental psychology. Developmental psychology complements several other basic research fields in psychology including social psychology, cognitive psychology, ecological psychology, and comparative psychology. What major problems face schools today and are likely to face them in the future? Nature of Educational Psychology, Human Growth and Development, Cognitive Development, Social, Emotional and Moral Development, Personality and Assessment and many more topics are competently dealt in this book.

— *Dr. Anamika*

Unit-I

Nature of Educational Psychology

Educational psychology has changed significantly over the 20th century. Early investigations of children as learners and the impact of different kinds of teaching approaches were largely characterized by attempts to identify general and consistent characteristics. The approaches used varied considerably. Jean Piaget, for example, recorded the development of individuals in detail, assessing changes with age and experience. Others, such as Robert Gagne, focused on the nature of teaching and learning, attempting to lay down taxonomies of learning outcomes. Alfred Binet and Cyril Burt were interested in methods of assessing children's development and identifying those children considered to be of high or low general intelligence.

This work led to productive research which refined the theories of development, learning, instruction, assessment, and evaluation, and built up an increasingly detailed picture of how students learn. Educational psychology became an essential part of the training of teachers, who for several generations were instructed in the theories emanating from its research to help train them in classroom teaching practice.

Changing Approaches

Recently the approach of educational psychology has changed significantly in the United Kingdom, as has its contribution to teacher education. In part these changes reflect political decisions to alter the pattern of teacher training: based on the belief that theory is not useful, and that "hands-on" training is preferable. However, discipline and teacher education have each been changing of their own accord. Moving away from the emphasis on all-encompassing theories, such as those of Jean Piaget, Sigmund Freud, and B. F. Skinner, the concerns of educational psychologists have shifted to practical issues and problems faced by the learner or the teacher. Consequently, rather than, for example, impart to teachers in training Skinner's theory of operant conditioning, and then seek ways of their applying it in classrooms, educational psychologists have tended to begin with the practical issues—how to teach reading; how to differentiate a curriculum (a planned course of teaching and learning) across a range of children with differing levels of achievement and needs; and how to manage discipline in classrooms. Theory-driven research increasingly suggested that more elaborated conceptions of development were required. For example, the earlier work on intelligence by Binet, Burt, and Lewis Madison Terman focused on the assessment of general intelligence, while recognizing that intellectual activity included verbal reasoning skills, general knowledge, and non-verbal abilities such as pattern recognition. More recently the emphasis has shifted to accentuate the differing profiles of abilities, or "multiple intelligences" as proposed by the American psychologist Howard Gardner, who argues that there is good evidence for at least seven, possibly more, intelligences including kinaesthetic and musical as well as the more traditionally valued linguistic and logico-mathematical types of intelligence.

There has also been a shift in emphasis from the student as an individual to the student in a social context, at all levels from specific cognitive (thinking and reasoning) abilities to general behaviour. For example, practical intelligence and its links with "common sense" have been addressed and investigations made into how individuals may have relatively low intelligence as measured by conventional intelligence tests, yet be seen to be highly intelligent in everyday tasks and "real-life" settings. Recognition of the impact of the environment on a child's general development has been informed by research on the effects of poverty, socio-economic status, gender, and cultural diversity, together with the effects of schooling itself. Also, the emphasis has changed from one of regarding differences in their performance on specific tasks as deficits compared with some norm, to an appreciation that deficits in performance may reflect unequal opportunity, or that differences may even reflect a positive diversity.

It is now apparent that there are also important biological factors determined by a child's genetic make-up and its prenatal existence, as well as social factors concerned with the family, school, and general social environment. Because these various factors all interact uniquely in the development of an individual, consequently there are limitations in the possible applicability of any one theory in educational psychology.

Definition of "Psychology"

The word "psychology" is the combination of two terms- study (ology) and soul (psyche), or mind. The derivation of the word from Latin gives it this clear and obvious meaning:

The study of the soul or mind.

This meaning has been altered over the years until today, this is not what the word means at all. The subject of psychology, as studied in colleges and universities, currently has very little to do with the mind, and absolutely nothing to do with the soul or spirit.

Let's see what a few dictionaries have to say and how a word could alter and lose it's true and actual meaning.

"Psyche" is defined as:

1. The spirit or soul.
2. The human mind.
3. In psychoanalysis, the mind functioning as the centre of thought, emotion, and behaviour.

And defining "soul", we have:

1. the spiritual or immortal elements in a person.
2. a person's mental or moral or emotional nature.

Most of us would agree we have a "psyche" per the above definitions in the sense of "mind", thought, and emotions. Most would also agree they have a "soul" per the second definition above relating to man's mental, moral or emotional nature. We might all have different notions about what these ultimately are, but few could sanely disagree they exist.

The derivation of "psyche" comes from Latin and the Greek *psukhe*-breath, life, soul. To get a better "feel" for this term think of it as the invisible animating principle or entity which occupies and directs the physical body.

We are not dealing with opinions or beliefs here. This is simply what the words and terms mean. Get clear on this first and understand what the words and terms mean, before you start getting into the opinions of others on the subject. If you choose to decide the "mind" refers to nothing real after understanding what the words and definitions mean, despite the fact that almost 10,000 years of thinking men have seriously and carefully looked into this subject, and after no real investigation on your own part, that's your decision. Also, realize you will be basing this decision on "thinking" and "reason", both of which are only subsidiary to and *part* of any one mind, and neglecting to use a greater aspect of your mind-your personal awareness and direct observation. Basing a decision on what other people say about a mind involves only *concepts* and *ideas* about a mind. Observation involves *experiencing the mind itself*-your own mind.

What is the Mind?

Originally, and for thousands of years, the subject of psychology involved the study of the human spirit, soul or mind. This involves things and functions not obviously visible to the physical senses. You can't see a mind with one's eyes. You can't "feel" a thought with one's hands. You can't place an emotion on a scale and weigh it. You can't detect imagination, even with sophisticated electronic detection devices. Modern "scientific" fields, since they haven't been able to study or detect these things with the physical senses or measuring devices have taken a drastic leap and declared that these things therefore don't exist, don't deserve recognition, and should be ignored in any "legitimate" study of man and the mind (and human behaviour). John Watson, a typical behavioural psychologist has this to say:

> *The extent to which most of us are shot through with a savage background is almost unbelievable.... One example of such a religious concept is that every individual has a soul which is separate and distinct from the body.... No one has ever touched a soul, or seen one in a test tube, or has in any way come into relationship with it as he has with the other objects of his daily experience....*
>
> *The behaviourist asks: Why don't we make what we can observe the real field of psychology? Let us limit ourselves to things that can be observed, and formulate laws concerning only those things. Now what can we observe? We can observe behaviour-what the organism does or says. And let us point out at once: that saying is doing-that is, behaving...-John Watson, behaviourist*

Strangely, the study of the mind has come into the peculiar position of being a study which denies the mind! That's like biology denying the existence of biological organisms, but going on pretending to still be the science of biological organisms while actually dealing with something else entirely. A subject can't exist if it denies the very basis of it's own existence by definition. That is the state of modern western psychology and psychiatry. Mmmm? They can't and shouldn't exist, but they do. The entire structure of these subjects as they currently exist is a sham.

Let's take a closer look at this. We each are quite aware we have a mind, emotions, and thoughts, even if we are not so clear or sure about the "soul" and "spirit". We know we are aware and possess self-awareness, but what the nature, qualities and potentials are of awareness is largely anybody's guess. We each know we possess consciousness. In fact, we are aware of our own consciousness as much or more than anything else, yet modern "science" ignores and even denies it. But the truth, despite what "science" or "professionals" say, is that the mind exists to and for each of us as an obvious and observable fact of direct experience. A quick look can tell us many obvious things. I doubt any of us would suggest we don't have a mind, awareness, thoughts or feelings even though none of these things can be detected or perceived with the physical senses or "scientific" measuring gadgets. *We don't immediately run off and deny their existence*, and we correctly assume others have similar minds, thoughts, feelings and emotions. They do. Modern psychologists and psychiatrists, for all practical purposes, completely deny every aspect of the invisible world known to you as your mind. It is invisible to physical detection, but it *does* exist.

There is constant activity within each of our "invisible worlds"-analyzing problems, entertaining thoughts of tomorrow's occurrences, recalling yesterday's failures, wallowing in the sadness of a loss, concentrating on the creation of a musical composition, day-dreaming, the ever-changing feelings and emotions about everything we experience, and the endless parade of judgments and commentary about what we see. Actually, for many of us, we have *too much* mind-it goes on and on, a constant source of images, memories and ideas intruding themselves upon our awareness. Most of us can't control any of this and simply accept as inevitable this continual parade of images and ideas across the landscape of our mind.

In a very real manner *all problems* with any mind, such as things psychiatry calls "depression", "anxiety", "compulsive disorder", "Attention Deficit Disorder" (ADD or ADHD), and even "suicidal ideation", are ultimately and solely *uncontrollable aspects of one's own mind which intrude upon the person's awareness*. It's not that these things don't exist in some way, but they don't exist in the way psychiatry understands and claims to solve them. A better way to handle these problems would be to assist the person to *increase control over the content of their own mind*. There are many ways to do this, although they have never been all pulled together, adequately investigated, codified and organized into a straight-forward workable compilation of methods. Modern "science" has simply discarded the notion of the mind, and from that point on, never bothered to investigate it closely with the aim to understand, solve or improve it.

First, this invisible world *is* totally real. It is *not* imaginary or a hallucination. My invisible world isn't directly real to you, and your invisible world isn't directly real to me, but they are *each real nonetheless*. The person who wants to argue this fact is simply a fool, dull, unable to comfortably observe his *own* mind (because it is possibly filled with degraded and evil things), and probably addicted to the objects of physical sensation and perception to the exclusion of everything else (a modern materialist). Second, this "invisible" world of mind involves many different aspects, functions and potentials. Imagination, attention, intellect, awareness, intention, reason, will, responsibility, memory, and many other things exist in each of us. They are a vital and important part of us-some might venture to say some of these things ARE us. There is much to each of these areas and a short essay cannot begin to even scratch the surface of their nature, functioning, possible development and capabilities. But they definitely *do exist* and deserve recognition and attention. Any subject calling itself "psychology" would have to address *these things* in detail. The failure of modern psychology and psychiatry to do so is glaringly apparent. These subjects now only address behaviour, physiology, genetics and biochemistry, and the mind is of no concern.

Methods in Psychology

As with most research, the study of developmental psychology begins with a **hypothesis**. A hypothesis is a testable statement that reflects what the researcher expects to find in a study. For example, a study on gender and learning disabilities might begin with a hypothesis that one gender will be more impacted by learning disorders. The goal of research is to analyze the area of interest, collect information and data about topic, draw conclusions based upon this research and data, and then add or expand upon previously existing theories of development.

Types of Research

There are a number of different ways to conduct psychological research. The two major types of research are:

1. **Cross-sectional Research:** Cross-sectional research involves looking at different groups of people of different ages. For example, a research might measure or observe a group of young adults and compare this data with information gathered about a group of elderly participants. The benefit of this type of research is that it can be done relatively quickly; the research data is all gathered at the same point in time. However, because data is gathered from generations of people who share the same cultural experiences, these shared events may play a role in development. This makes it difficult to determine if something is caused by experience or the aging process.
2. **Longitudinal Research:** Longitudinal research involves studying the same group of individuals over an extended period of time. Data is first collected at the outset of the study, and may then be gathered repeatedly throughout the length of the study. In some cases, longitudinal studies can last several decades. The benefit of this type of research is that it allows researchers to look at changes over time. However, longitudinal studies require enormous amounts of time and are often quite expensive. Because of this, these studies often have only a small group of subjects, which makes it difficult to apply the results to a larger population. Another problem is that participants sometimes drop out of the study, shrinking the sample size and decreasing the amount of data collected.

Data Collection

Once it has been decided which type of research to use, the next step is to determine how the information will be gathered.

There are a number of different research methods that are used in the study of developmental psychology, each with its own strengths and weaknesses. Some common approaches include observation, case studies, questionnaires, and experimentation.

Observation

There are two different types of observation. The first involves viewing the subject of interest in a laboratory setting. The benefit of this is that the situation can be controlled by the experimental. The drawbacks of lab observation are that the setting can be unnatural and the subject is aware that they are being studied. Both of these factors can have an impact on results of the study. Naturalistic observation allows researchers to observe participants in real-world settings. The strength of this method is that it allows researchers to view behaviour as it really happens in a natural setting. The drawback is that the researcher cannot control outside variables that might impact behaviour.

Case Studies

A case study is an in-depth analysis of a particular individual. While this research method provides a great deal of information about a specific person, the results are often difficult to generalize to larger populations. For this reason, case studies are most often used in clinical research or other cases where certain aspects of the subject's life cannot be reproduced or duplicated.

Questionnaires

Questionnaires offer researchers a quick, easy way to collect a great deal of information. One weakness of this method is that it reduces variety, creativity, and individuality of responses. In cases where the subject is unable to fill out a questionnaire, with very young children for example, questions are often posed through a structured interview.

Experimentation

Experiments involve the manipulation and measurement of variables. This research method is the most scientific, but it can be difficult to use if the variables of interest are abstract or internal concepts. Another problem is that some variables of interest cannot be studied through experimentation for ethical reasons. Examples of this would be research on the effects of child abuse on development.

Branches of Psychology

Overview of the Major Branches of Psychology

There are a number of unique and distinctive branches of psychology. Each branch looks at questions and problems from a different perspective. While each branch has its own focus on psychological problems or concerns, all areas share a common goal of studying and explaining human thought and behaviour. The following are some of the major branches of psychology within the field today.

1. **Abnormal Psychology:** Abnormal psychology is the branch of psychology that looks at psychopathology and abnormal behaviour. The term covers a broad range of disorders, from depression to obsession-compulsion to sexual deviation and many more. Counsellors, clinical psychologists, and psychotherapists often work directly in this field.
2. **Behavioural Psychology:** Behavioural psychology, also known as behaviourism, is a theory of learning based upon the idea that all behaviours are acquired through conditioning. While this branch of psychology dominated the field during the first part of the twentieth century, its hold loosened during the 1950s. However, Behavioural techniques remain a mainstay in therapy, education and many other areas.
3. **Biopsychology:** The branch of psychology focused on the study of how the brain influences behaviour is often known as biopsychology, although it has also been called physiological psychology, Behavioural neuroscience and psychobiology.
4. **Cognitive Psychology:** Cognitive psychology is the branch of psychology that focuses on internal states, such as motivation, problem solving, decision-making, thinking, and attention. This area of psychology has continued to grow since it began taking hold in the 1960s.
5. **Comparative Psychology:** Comparative psychology is the branch of psychology concerned with the study

of animal behaviour. The study of animal behaviour can lead to a deeper and broader understanding of human psychology.

6. **Developmental Psychology:** This branch of psychology looks at development throughout the lifespan, from childhood to adulthood. The scientific study of human development seeks to understand and explain how and why people change throughout life. This includes all aspects of human growth, including physical, emotional, intellectual, social, perceptual, and personality development. Topics studied in this field include everything from prenatal development to Alzheimer's disease.
7. **Educational Psychology:** Educational psychology is the branch of psychology concerned with schools, teaching psychology, educational issues, and student concerns. Educational psychologists often study how students learn or work directly with students, parents, teachers and administrators to improve student outcomes.
8. **Experimental Psychology:** Experimental psychology is the branch of psychology that utilizes scientific methods to research the brain and behaviour. Many of these techniques are also used by other areas in psychology to conduct research on everything from childhood development to social issues.
9. **Personality Psychology:** This branch of psychology is focused on the patterns of thoughts, feelings, and behaviour that make a person unique. Some of the best-known theories in psychology have arisen from this field, including Freud's stage theory of psychosexual development and Erikson's theory of psychosocial development.
10. **Social Psychology:** Social psychology seeks to explain and understand social behaviour and looks at diverse topics including group behaviour. social interactions, leadership, nonverbal communication and social influences on decision-making.

Educational Psychology: Definition

Educational psychology is the study of how humans learn in educational settings, the effectiveness of educational interventions, the psychology of teaching, and the social psychology of schools as organizations. Although the terms "educational psychology" and "school psychology" are often used interchangeably, In the US researchers and theorists are likely to be identified as educational psychologists, whereas practitioners in schools or school-related settings are identified as school psychologists. In the UK, however, this distinction is not made and the generic term for practitioners is "Educational Psychologist." Educational psychology is concerned with how students learn and develop, often focusing on subgroups such as gifted children and those subject to specific disabilities.

Educational psychology can in part be understood through its relationship with other disciplines. It is informed primarily by psychology, bearing a relationship to that discipline analogous to the relationship between medicine and biology and also between Engineering and Physics. Educational psychology in turn informs a wide range of specialities within educational studies, including instructional design, educational technology, curriculum development, organizational learning, special education and classroom management. Educational psychology both draws from and contributes to cognitive science and the learning sciences. In universities, departments of educational psychology are usually housed within faculties of education, possibly accounting for the lack of representation of educational psychology content in introductory psychology textbooks.

Nature and Scope of Educational Psychology

In this age of science and technology, psychology has been considered as one of the youngest, yet one of the most influential sciences. It has influenced education in many different ways and has give a new turn; a psychological turn to the human mind. For a skilful teacher in this day and age, a great deal of knowledge of educational psychology is highly indispensable.

The subject psychology has two aspects pure and applied. Pure psychology formulates techniques for the study of human behaviour, which finds the practical shape in its applied aspects, i.e. branches of applied psychology like clinical psychology, crime psychology, industrial psychology, occupational psychology and educational psychology. Educational Psychology as a Branch of Applied Psychology.

As discussed above educational psychology is nothing but one of the branches of applied psychology. It is an attempt to apply knowledge of pure psychology to the field of education. It consists of application of psychological principles and techniques to human behaviour in educational situations. In other words, Educational Psychology is a study of the experience and behaviour of the learner in relation to educational environment. In order to develop a clear understanding of the term educational psychology it is necessary to understand the meaning of psychology and education separately.

Meaning of Psychology

Curiosity in man has led to know his surroundings which mainly conclude nature and other fellow men. There is always a desire to 'know' what 'one' is, what is his background, what is it made of, what are the associated factors and in what way can it be useful to one self? Each question will lead to more questions, Psychology forces to answer many of the questions we have about ourselves, other people and the nature of human life; why do we feel lonely? Why do we forget? How people learn? What makes someone creative? Why do we take drugs? What makes some one help others? and so on.

Psychology had its formal beginning when Wilhelm Wondt established his psychological laboratory in Leipzig Germany in 1879. But in real sense, interest in psychology as a discipline dates back to the work of Plato, Aristotle and other philosophers.

Psychology – The Science of Soul

The Greek Philosophers conceived psychology as a science of soul, as early as 400 B.C. In fact, the term psychology literally means the science of soul. Etymologically, it is composed of two Greek words "Psyche" and Logos means soul and science respectively. Goeckel named it as psychologia. Soul is a being which dwells on the body and with the end of life it leaves the body. Soul is a metaphysical idea. It can neither be perceived on imagined nor its nature and function can be studied by scientific methods of observation, experiment etc. Therefore, definition of psychology as the science of soul has been discarded by the modern psychologists.

Psychology – The Science of Mind

Some regard psychology as the science of mind. Historically the French philosophers like Descartes (1596-1650) and the Britisher philosophers like Locke considered psychology as the science of mind. Descartes tried to understand body mind relationship in terms of their interaction, the study of nervous system, and interest of references as innate actions, etc. The definition of psychology as the science of mind is not acceptable at present. Mind is an ambiguous a concept as the soul. It is not at all possible to carry on scientific observation and experimentation on mind. This definition also does not include the overt behaviour of man and animal which are also important subject matter of psychology. Therefore, the definition of psychology as the science of mind has been discarded.

Psychology – The Science of Consciousness

Psychology has also been defined as the science of consciousness. Historically such a definition has been propounded by the Leipzing school of psychologists led by Withelm Wundt (1832-1920). Wundt defined psychology as the science of immediate experience with consciousness being the main subject matter. He postulated that conscious experience can be reduced in to elements and the primary aim psychology is the analysis of conscious experience in to its elements. But the definition of psychology as the science of consciousness is not acceptable. That is because mental life does not consist only of consciousness. There are unconscious and subconscious mental process which influence our behaviour in various ways without our knowledge.

Psychology – The Science of Experience

Titchner (1867 – 1927), the leader of the structuralists defines psychology as the science of conscious experience which is dependent upon the experiencing person. To give an example the physicit and the psychologist may be investigating about sound. But whole the former investigates the phenomena as such, the latter is interested as to how it is perceived by the observer. The mind is nothing but the sum total of the conscious experiences as perceived by a person. The subject matter of psychology is the study of such conscious experience which constitutes mind. The method of study of conscious experience is through the introspection of a trained observer.

Psychology – Study of Behaviour

Watson (1878-1958), an American brought about a revolution in psychology called behaviourism. He argued that psychology is to be regarded as a science and as a science it is to limit itself to the study and analysis of publicly observable events such as the behaviour of the subject rather than subjective matters like his private mental states. He defined psychology as "the science of behaviour."

Meaning of Science and Behaviour

Science has been defined as "Systematic study of knowledge" concerning the relationship between the cause and effect of a particular phenomenon. In order to collect the scientific data and systematised material, science employs various kinds of methods of enquiry such as observation classification formulation of hypothesis, analysis of evidence etc. It also organises and develops our knowledge of the word, we live on, Psychology too aims at same thing. It uses scientific methods to study human behaviour. It also helps us to understand control and predict human behaviour.

What is Social Learning Theory?

The social learning theory proposed by Albert Bandura has become perhaps the most influential theory of learning and development. While rooted in many of the basic concepts of traditional learning theory, Bandura believed that direct reinforcement could not account for all types of learning.

His theory added a social element, arguing that people can learn new information and behaviours by watching other people.

Known as observational learning (or modelling), this type of learning can be used to explain a wide variety of behaviours.

Basic Social Learning Concepts

1. People can learn through observation.

Observational Learning

In his famous "Bobo doll" studies, Bandura demonstrated that children learn and imitate behaviours they have observed in other people. The children in Bandura's studies observed an adult acting violently toward a Bobo doll. When the children were later allowed to play in a room with the Bobo doll, they began to imitate the aggressive actions they had previously observed.

Bandura identified three basic models of observational learning:

1. A live model, which involves an actual individual demonstrating or acting out a behaviour.
2. A verbal instructional model, which involves descriptions and explanations of a behaviour.
3. A symbolic model, which involves real or fictional characters displaying behaviours in books, films, television programs, or online media.

2. *Mental states are important to learning.*

Intrinsic Reinforcement

Bandura noted that external, environmental reinforcement was not the only factor to influence learning and behaviour. He described intrinsic reinforcement as a form of internal reward, such as pride, satisfaction, and a sense of accomplishment.

This emphasis on internal thoughts and cognitions helps connect learning theories to cognitive developmental theories. While many textbooks place social learning theory with Behavioural theories, Bandura himself describes his approach as a 'social cognitive theory.'

3. *Learning does not necessarily lead to a change in behaviour.*

While behaviourists believed that learning led to a permanent change in behaviour, observational learning demonstrates that people can learn new information without demonstrating new behaviours.

The Modelling Process

Not all observed behaviours are effectively learned. Factors involving both the model and the learner can play a role in whether social learning is successful. Certain requirements and steps must also be followed.

The following steps are involved in the observational learning and Modelling process:

- **Attention:** In order to learn, you need to be paying attention. Anything that detracts your attention is going to have a negative effect on observational learning. If the model interesting or there is a novel aspect to the situation, you are far more likely to dedicate your full attention to learning.
- **Retention:** The ability to store information is also an important part of the learning process. Retention can be affected by a number of factors, but the ability to pull up information later and act on it is vital to observational learning.
- **Reproduction:** Once you have paid attention to the model and retained the information, it is time to actually perform the behaviour you observed. Further practice of the learned behaviour leads to improvement and skill advancement.
- **Motivation:** Finally, in order for observational learning to be successful, you have to be motivated to imitate the behaviour that has been modelled. Reinforcement and punishment play an important role in motivation. While experiencing these motivators can be highly effective, so can observing other experience some type of reinforcement or punishment. For example, if you see another student rewarded with extra credit for being to class on time, you might start to show up a few minutes early each day.

Why Classroom Management Matters?

Managing the learning environment is both a major responsibility and an on-going concern for every teacher, even those with years of experience (Good & Brophy, 2002). There are several reasons. In the first place, a lot goes on in classrooms simultaneously, even when students seem to be doing only "one" task together. Twenty-five students may all be working on a sheet of math problems. But look more closely: several may be stuck on a particular problem, but each for different reasons. A few others have worked only the first problem or two and are now chatting quietly with each other instead of continuing. Still others have finished and are wondering what to do next. At any one moment each student needs something different—different information, different hints, different kinds of encouragement. The diversity increases even more if the teacher deliberately assigns multiple activities to different groups or individuals (for example, if some are doing a reading assignment while others do the math problems).

Another reason that managing the environment is challenging is because a teacher can never predict everything that will happen in a class. A well-planned lesson may fall flat on its face, or take less time than you expect, and you find yourself improvising to fill class time. On the other hand an unplanned moment may become a wonderful, sustained exchange among students; so you have to drop previous plans and "go with the flow" of their discussion. Interruptions happen continually: a fire drill, a quick drop-in visit from another teacher or from the principal, a call on the intercom from the office. An activity may turn out well, but also end up rather differently than you intended; you therefore have to decide how, if at all, to adjust the next day to allow for this surprise.

A third reason for the importance of management is that students form opinions and perceptions about your teaching that may coincide neither with your own nor with other students'. What seems to you like encouragement of a shy student may seem to the student herself like "forced participation." A more eager, outgoing classmate watching your special effort to encourage the shy student, however, may not see you as either encouraging or coercing, but as overlooking or ignoring other students who are already more willing to participate. The variety of perceptions can lead to surprises in students' responses to you—most often small ones, but occasionally more major.

At the broadest, society-wide level, management challenges teachers because public schooling is not voluntary, and students' presence in a classroom is therefore not a sign, in and of itself, that they wish to learn. Students' presence is instead just a sign that an opportunity exists for teachers to motivate students to learn. Many students, of course, do enjoy learning and being in school—but not all. Others do enjoy school, but primarily because teachers have worked hard to make classroom life pleasant and interesting. They become motivated because you have successfully created a positive learning environment and have sustained it through skilful management.

Fortunately it is possible to earn this sort of commitment from students, and this chapter describes some ways of doing so. We begin with some ways of preventing management problems in the first place by increasing students' focus on learning. The methods include the arrangement of classroom space, the establishment of procedures, routines, and rules, and communicating the importance of learning both to students and to parents. After these prevention oriented discussions, we look at ways of refocusing students when and if their minds or actions do stray from the tasks at hand. As you probably know from your own experience as a student, bringing students back on task can happen in many ways, ways that vary widely in the energy and persistence required of the teacher. We try to indicate some of this diversity, but because of space limitations and because of the richness of classroom life, we cannot describe them all.

Learner

Learning is acquiring new knowledge, behaviours, skills, values, preferences or understanding, and may involve synthesizing different types of information. The ability to learn is possessed by humans, animals and some machines. Progress over time tends to follow learning curves. Human learning may occur as part of education or personal development. It may be goal-oriented and may be aided by motivation. The study of how learning occurs is part of neuropsychology, educational psychology, learning theory, and pedagogy.

Learning may occur as a result of habituation or classical conditioning, seen in many animal species, or as a result of more complex activities such as play, seen only in relatively intelligent animals and humans. Learning may occur consciously or without conscious awareness. There is evidence for human behavioural learning prenatally, in which habituation has been observed as early as 32 weeks into gestation, indicating that the central nervous system is sufficiently developed and primed for learning and memory to occur very early on in development.

Play has been approached by several theorists as the first form of learning. Children play, experiment with the world, learn the rules, and learn to interact. Vygotsky agrees that play is pivotal for children's development, since they make meaning of their environment through play.

Learning Process

To learn is to acquire knowledge or skill. Learning also may involve a change in attitude or behaviour. Children learn to identify objects at an early age; teenagers may learn to improve study habits; and adults can learn to solve complex problems. Pilots and aviation maintenance technicians (AMTs) need to acquire the higher levels of knowledge and skill, including the ability to exercise judgment and solve problems. The challenge for the aviation instructor is to understand how people learn, and more importantly, to be able to apply that knowledge to the learning environment. This handbook is designed as a basic guide to educational psychology. This chapter addresses that branch of psychology directly concerned with how people learn.

Learning Theory

Learning theory may be described as a body of principles advocated by psychologists and educators to explain how people acquire skills, knowledge, and attitudes. Various branches of learning theory are used in formal training programs to improve and accelerate the learning process. Key concepts such as desired learning outcomes, objectives of the training, and depth of training also apply. When properly integrated, learning principles, derived from theories, can be useful to aviation instructors and developers of instructional programs for both pilots and maintenance technicians.

Over the years, many theories have attempted to explain how people learn. Even though psychologists and educators are not in complete agreement, most do agree that learning may be explained by a combination of two basic approaches: behaviourism and the cognitive theories.

Behaviourism

Behaviourists believe that animals, including humans, learn in about the same way. Behaviourism stresses the importance of having a particular form of behaviour reinforced by someone, other than the student, to shape or control what is learned. In aviation training, the instructor provides the reinforcement. Frequent, positive reinforcement and rewards accelerate learning. This theory provides the instructor with ways to manipulate students with stimuli, induce the desired behaviour or response, and reinforce the behaviour with appropriate rewards. In general, the behaviourist theory emphasizes positive reinforcement rather than no reinforcement or punishment. Other features of behaviourism are considerably more complex than this simple explanation. Instructors who need more details should refer to psychology texts for a better understanding of behaviourism. As an instructor, it is important to keep in mind that behaviourism is still widely used today, because controlling learning experiences helps direct students toward specific learning outcomes.

Cognitive Theory

Much of the recent psychological thinking and experimentation in education includes some facets of the cognitive theory. This is true in basic as well as more advanced training programs. Unlike behaviourism, the cognitive theory focuses on what is going on inside the student's mind. Learning is not just a change in behaviour; it is a change in the way a student thinks, understands, or feels.

There are several branches of cognitive theory. Two of the major theories may broadly be classified as the information processing model and the social interaction model. The first says that the student's brain has internal structures which select and process incoming material, store and retrieve it, use it to produce behaviour, and receive and process feedback on the results.

This involves a number of cognitive processes, including executive functions of recognizing expectancies, planning and monitoring performance, encoding and chunking information, and producing internal and external responses.

The social interaction theories gained prominence in the 1980s. They stress that learning and subsequent changes in behaviour take place as a result of interaction between the student and the environment. Behaviour is modelled either by people or symbolically. Cultural influences, peer pressure, group dynamics, and film and television are some of the significant factors. Thus, the social environment to which the student is exposed demonstrates or models behaviours, and the student cognitively processes the observed behaviours and consequences. The cognitive processes include attention, retention, motor responses, and motivation. Techniques for learning include direct modelling and verbal instruction. Behaviour, personal factors, and environmental events all work together to produce learning.

Both models of the cognitive theory have common principles. For example, they both acknowledge the importance of reinforcing behaviour and measuring changes. Positive reinforcement is important, particularly with cognitive concepts such as knowledge and understanding. The need to evaluate and measure behaviour remains because it is the only way to get a clue about what the student understands. Evaluation is often limited to the kinds of knowledge or behaviour that can be measured by a paper-and-pencil exam or a performance test. Although psychologists agree that there often are errors in evaluation, some means of measuring student knowledge, performance, and behaviour is necessary.

Combined Approach

Both the behaviouristic and the cognitive approaches are useful learning theories. A reasonable way to plan, manage, and conduct aviation training is to include the best features of each major theory. This provides a way to measure behavioural outcomes and promote cognitive learning. The combined approach is not simple, but neither is learning.

Definition of Learning

The ability to learn is one of the most outstanding human characteristics. Learning occurs continuously throughout a person's lifetime. To define learning, it is necessary to analyze what happens to the individual. For example, an individual's way of perceiving, thinking, feeling, and doing may change as a result of a learning experience. Thus, learning can be defined as a change in behaviour as a result of experience. This can be physical and overt, or it may involve complex intellectual or attitudinal changes which affect behaviour in more subtle ways. In spite of numerous theories and contrasting views, psychologists generally agree on many common characteristics of learning.

Characteristics of Learning

Learning is Purposeful: Each student sees a learning situation from a different viewpoint. Each student is a unique individual whose past experiences affect readiness to learn and understanding of the requirements involved. For example, an instructor may give two aviation maintenance students the assignment of learning certain inspection procedures. One student may learn quickly and be able to competently present the assigned material. The combination of an aviation background and future goals may enable that student to realize the need and value of learning the procedures. A second student's goal may only be to comply with the instructor's assignment, and may result in only minimum preparation. The responses differ because each student ads in accordance with what he or she sees in the situation. Most people have fairly definite ideas about what they want to do and achieve. Their goals sometimes are short term, involving a matter of days or weeks. On the other hand, their goals may be carefully planned for a career or a lifetime. Each student has specific intentions and goals. Some may be shared by other students. Students learn from any activity that tends to further their goals. Their individual needs and attitudes may determine what they learn as much as what the instructor is trying to get them to learn. In the process of learning, the student's goals are of paramount significance. To be effective, aviation instructors need to find ways to relate new learning to the student's goals.

Learning is a Result of Experience

Since learning is an individual process, the instructor cannot do it for the student. The student can learn only from personal experiences; therefore, learning and knowledge cannot exist apart from a person. A person's knowledge is a result of experience, and no two people have had identical experiences. Even when observing the same event, two people react differently; they learn different things from it, according to the manner in which the situation affects their individual needs. Previous experience conditions a person to respond to some things and to ignore others.

All learning is by experience, but learning takes place in different forms and in varying degrees of richness and depth. For instance, some experiences involve the whole person while others may be based only on hearing and memory. Aviation instructors are faced with the problem of providing learning experiences that are meaningful, varied, and appropriate. As an example, students can learn to say a list of words through repeated drill, or they can learn to recite certain principles of flight by rote. However, they can make them meaningful only if they understand them well enough to apply them correctly to real situations. If an experience challenges the students, requires involvement with feelings, thoughts, memory of past experiences, and physical activity, it is more effective than a learning experience in which all the students have to do is commit something to memory.

It seems clear enough that the learning of a physical skill requires actual experience in performing that skill. Student pilots learn to fly aircraft only if their experiences include flying them; student aviation maintenance technicians learn to overhaul powerplants only by actually performing that task. Mental habits are also learned through practice. If students are to use sound judgment and develop decision-making skills, they need learning experiences that involve knowledge of general principles and require the use of judgment in salving realistic problems.

Learning is Multifaceted

If instructors see their objective as being only to train their students' memory and muscles, they are underestimating the potential of the teaching situation. Students may learn much more than expected if they fully exercise their minds and feelings. The fact that these items were not included in the instructor's plan does not prevent them from influencing the learning situation.

Psychologists sometimes classify learning by types, such as verbal, conceptual, perceptual, motor, problem solving, and emotional. Other classifications refer to intellectual skills, cognitive strategies, and attitudinal changes, along with descriptive terms like surface or deep learning. However useful these divisions may be, they are somewhat artificial. For example, a class learning to apply the scientific method of problem solving may learn the method by trying to solve real problems. But in doing so, the class also engages in verbal learning and sensory perception at the same time. Each student approaches the task with preconceived ideas and feelings, and for many students, these ideas change as a result of experience. Therefore, the learning process may include verbal elements, conceptual elements, perceptual elements, emotional elements, and problem solving elements all taking place at once. This aspect of learning will become more evident later in this handbook when lesson planning is discussed.

Learning is multifaceted in still another way. While learning the subject at hand, students may be learning other things as well. They may be developing attitudes about aviation-good or bad-depending on what they experience. Under a skilful instructor, they may learn self-reliance. The list is seemingly endless. This type of learning is sometimes referred to as incidental, but it may have a great impact on the total development of the student.

Learning is an Active Process

Students do not soak up knowledge like a sponge absorbs water. The instructor cannot assume that students remember something just because they were in the classroom, shop, or airplane when the instructor presented the material. Neither can the instructor assume that the students can apply what they know because they can quote the correct answer verbatim. For students to learn, they need to react and respond, perhaps outwardly, perhaps only inwardly, emotionally, or intellectually. But if learning is a process of changing behaviour, clearly that process must be an active one.

Learning Styles

Although characteristics of learning and learning styles are related, there are distinctions between the two. Learning style is a concept that can play an important role in improving instruction and student success. It is concerned with student preferences and orientation at several levels. For example, a student's information processing technique, personality, social interaction tendencies and the instructional methods used are all significant factors which apply to how individual students learn. In addition, today's culturally diverse society, including international students, must be considered.

The key point is that all students are different, and training programs should be sensitive to the differences. Some students are fast learners and others have difficulties; and, as already mentioned, motivation, experience, and previous training affect learning style. Any number of adjectives may be used to describe learning styles. Some common examples include:

- Right/left brain
- Holistic/serialist

- Dependent/independent
- Reflective/impulsive

Theories abound concerning right- or left-brain dominance. In general, those with right-brain dominance are characterized as being spatially oriented, creative, intuitive, and emotional. Those with left-brain dominance are more verbal, analytical, and objective. However, the separate hemispheres of the brain do not function independently. For example, the right hemisphere may recognize a face, while the left associates a name to go with the face. The term dominance is probably misleading when applied to brain hemispheres; specialization would be a more appropriate word.

Learning style differences certainly depend on how students process information. Some rely heavily on visual references while others depend more on auditory presentations. For example, visual students learn readily through reading and graphic displays, and auditory students have more success if they hear the subject matter described. Another difference is that some learn more easily when an idea is presented in a mathematical equation, while others may prefer a verbal explanation of the same idea. In addition, where hands-on activities are involved, students also learn by feel. This is sometimes called kinesthetic learning. Information processing theories contain several other useful classifications. As an example, in the holistic/serialist theory, the holist strategy is a top-down concept where students have a big picture, global perspective. These students seek overall comprehension, especially through the use of analogies. In contrast, the serialist student focuses more narrowly and needs well-defined, sequential steps where the overall picture is developed slowly, thoroughly, and logically. This is a bottom-up strategy.

Two additional information processing classifications describe deep-elaborative and the shallow-reiterative learners. Testing practices which demand comprehension, rather than a regurgitation of facts, obviously encourage students to adopt a deep-elaborative learning style. Detailed information on testing procedures, as well as curriculum design and instructor techniques, is included later in this handbook.

As indicated, personality also affects how students learn. Dependent students require a lot of guidance, direction, and external stimulation. These students tend to focus on the instructor. The more independent students require only a minimum amount of guidance and external stimulation. They are not overly concerned with how the lesson is presented.

Students with a reflective-type personality may be described as tentative. They tend to be uncertain in problem-solving exercises. The opposite applies to impulsive students. Typically, they dive right in with enthusiasm and are prone to make quick, and sometimes faulty, decisions.

The social interaction concept contains further classifications of student learning styles. Like most of the other information on learning styles, these classifications are derived from research on tendencies of undergraduate students.

Some generalizations about these classifications indicate that compliant students are typically task oriented, and anxious-dependent students usually score lower than others on standardized tests. Discouraged students often have depressed feelings about the future, and independent students tend to be older, intelligent, secure, and comfortable with the academic environment. Attention seekers have a strong social orientation and are frequently involved in joking, showing off, and bragging. In contrast, silent students usually are characterized by helplessness, vulnerability, and other disconcerting behaviourism.

Other studies identify more categories that are easily recognized. Among these are collaborative, sharing students who enjoy working with others, and competitive students who are grade conscious and feel they must do better than their peers. Participant students normally have a desire to learn and enjoy attending class, and avoidant students do not take part in class activities and have little interest in learning.

The existing learning environment also influences learning style. In real life, most students find it necessary to adapt to a traditional style learning environment provided by a school, university, or other educational/training establishment. Thus, the student's learning style may or may not be compatible.

Instructors who can recognize student learning style differences and associated problems will be much more effective than those who do not understand this concept. Also, these instructors will be prepared to develop appropriate lesson plans and provide guidance, counselling, or other advisory services, as required.

Principles of Learning

Over the years, educational psychologists have identified several principles which seem generally applicable to the learning process. They provide additional insight into what makes people learn most effectively.

Readiness

Individuals learn best when they are ready to learn, and they do not learn well if they see no reason for learning. Getting students ready to learn is usually the instructor's responsibility. If students have a strong purpose, a clear objective, and a definite reason for learning something, they make more progress than if they lack motivation. Readiness implies a degree of single-mindedness and eagerness. When students are ready to learn, they meet the instructor at least halfway, and this simplifies the instructor's job.

Under certain circumstances, the instructor can do little, if anything, to inspire in students a readiness to learn. If outside responsibilities, interests, or worries weigh too heavily on their minds, if their schedules are overcrowded, or if their personal problems seem insoluble, students may have little interest in learning.

Exercise

The principle of exercise states that those things most often repeated are best remembered. It is the basis of drill and practice. The human memory is fallible. The mind can rarely retain, evaluate, and apply new concepts or practices after a single exposure. Students do not learn to weld during one shop period or to perform crosswise landings during one instructional flight. They learn by applying what they have been told and shown. Every time practice occurs, learning continues. The instructor must provide opportunities for students to practice and, at the same time, make sure that this process is directed toward a goal.

Effect

The principle of effect is based on the emotional reaction of the student. It states that learning is strengthened when accompanied by a pleasant or satisfying feeling, and that learning is weakened when associated with an unpleasant feeling. Experiences that produce feelings of defeat, frustration, anger, confusion, or futility are unpleasant for the student. If, for example, an instructor attempts to teach landings during the first flight, the student is likely to feel inferior and be frustrated.

Instructors should be cautious. Impressing students with the difficulty of an aircraft maintenance problem, flight manoeuvre or flight crew duty can make the teaching task difficult. Usually it is better to tell students that a problem or manoeuvre, although difficult, is within their capability to understand or perform. Whatever the learning situation, it should contain elements that affect the students positively and give them a feeling of satisfaction.

Primacy

Primacy, the state of being first, often creates a strong, almost unshakable, impression. For the instructor, this means that what is taught must be right the first time. For the student, it means that learning must be right. Unteaching is more difficult than teaching. If, for example, a maintenance student learns a faulty riveting technique, the instructor will have a difficult task correcting bad habits and reteaching correct ones. Every student should be started right. The first experience should be positive, functional, and lay the foundation for all that is to follow.

Intensity

A vivid, dramatic, or exciting learning experience teaches more than a routine or boring experience. A student is likely to gain greater understanding of slow flight and stalls by performing them rather than merely reading about them. The principle of intensity implies that a student will learn more from the real thing than from a substitute. In contrast to flight instruction and shop instruction, the classroom imposes limitations on the amount of realism that can be brought into teaching. The aviation instructor should use imagination in approaching reality as closely as possible. Today, classroom instruction can benefit from a wide variety of instructional aids to improve realism, motivate learning, and challenge students. Chapter 7, Instructional Aids and Training Technologies, explores the wide range of teaching tools available for classroom use.

Recency

The principle of recency states that things most recently learned are best remembered. Conversely, the further a student is removed time-wise from a new fact or understanding, the more difficult it is to remember. It is easy, for example, for a student to recall a torque value used a few minutes earlier, but it is usually impossible to remember an unfamiliar one used a week earlier. Instructors recognize the principle of recency when they carefully plan a summary for a ground school lesson, a shop period, or a postflight critique. The instructor repeats, restates, or reemphasizes important points at the end of a lesson to help the student remember them. The principle of recency often determines the sequence of lectures within a course of instruction.

How People Learn?

Perceptions: Perceiving involves more than the reception of stimuli from the five senses. Perceptions result when a person gives meaning to sensations. People base their actions on the way they believe things to be. The experienced aviation maintenance technician, for example, perceives an engine malfunction quite differently than does an inexperienced student. Real meaning comes only from within a person, even though the perceptions which evoke these meanings result from external stimuli. The meanings which are derived from perceptions are influenced not only by the individual's experience, but also by many other factors. Knowledge of the factors which affect the perceptual process is very important to the aviation instructor because perceptions are the basis of all learning.

Factors which Affect Perception

There are several factors that affect an individual's ability to perceive. Some are internal to each person and some are external.

- Physical organism
- Basic need
- Goals and values
- Self-concept
- Time and opportunity
- Element of threat

Physical Organism

The physical organism provides individuals with the perceptual apparatus for sensing the world around them. Pilots, for example, must be able to see, hear, feel, and respond adequately while they are in the air. A person whose perceptual apparatus distorts reality is denied the right to fly at the time of the first medical examination.

Basic Need

A person's basic need is to maintain and enhance the organized self. The self is a person's past, present, and future combined; it is both physical and psychological. A person's most fundamental, pressing need is to preserve and perpetuate the self. All perceptions are affected by this need.

Just as the food one eats and the air one breathes become part of the physical self, so do the sights one sees and the sounds one hears become part of the psychological self. Psychologically, we are what we perceive. A person has physical barriers which keep out those things that would be damaging to the physical being, such as blinking at an arc weld or flinching from a hot iron. Likewise, a person has perceptual barriers that block those sights, sounds, and feelings which pose a psychological threat. Helping people learn requires finding ways to aid them in developing better perceptions in spite of their defense mechanisms. Since a person's basic need is to maintain and enhance the self, the instructor must recognize that anything that is asked of the student which may be interpreted by the student as imperilling the self will be resisted or denied. To teach effectively, it is necessary to work with this life force.

Goals and Values

Perceptions depend on one's goals and values. Every experience and sensation which is funnelled into one's central nervous system is coloured by the individual's own beliefs and value structures. Spectators at a ball game may see an infraction or foul differently depending on which team they support. The precise kinds of commitments and philosophical outlooks which the student holds are important for the instructor to know, since this knowledge will assist in predicting how the student will interpret experiences and instructions.

Goals are also a product of one's value structure. Those things which are more highly valued and cherished are pursued; those which are accorded less value and importance are not sought after.

Self-Concept

Self-concept is a powerful determinant in learning. A student's self-image, described in such terms as confident and insecure, has a great influence on the total perceptual process. If a student's experiences tend to support a favourable self-image, the student tends to remain receptive to subsequent experiences. If a student has negative experiences which tend to contradict self-concept, there is a tendency to reject additional training.

A negative self-concept inhibits the perceptual processes by introducing psychological barriers which tend to keep the student from perceiving. They may also inhibit the ability to properly implement that which is perceived. That is, self-concept affects the ability to actually perform or do things unfavourable. Students who view themselves positively, on the other hand, are less defensive and more receptive to new experiences, instructions, and demonstrations.

Time and Opportunity

It takes time and opportunity to perceive. Learning some things depends on other perceptions which have preceded these learnings, and on the availability of time to sense and relate these new things to the earlier perceptions. Thus, sequence and time are necessary.

A student could probably stall an airplane on the first attempt, regardless of previous experience. Stalls cannot really be learned, however, unless some experience in normal flight has been acquired. Even with such experience, time and practice are needed to relate the new sensations and experiences associated with stalls in order to develop a perception of the stall. In general, lengthening an experience and increasing its frequency are the most obvious ways to speed up learning, although this is not always effective. Many factors, in addition to the length and frequency of training periods, affect the rate of learning. The effectiveness of the use of a properly planned training syllabus is proportional to the consideration it gives to the time and opportunity factor in perception.

Element of Threat

The element of threat does not promote effective learning. In fact, fear adversely affects perception by narrowing the perceptual field. Confronted with threat, students tend to limit their attention to the threatening object or condition. The field of vision is reduced, for example, when an individual is frightened and all the perceptual faculties are focused on the thing that has generated fear.

Flight instruction provides many clear examples of this. During the initial practice of steep turns, a student pilot may focus attention on the altimeter and completely disregard outside visual references. Anything an instructor does that is interpreted as threatening makes the student less able to accept the experience the instructor is trying to provide. It adversely affects all the student's physical, emotional, and mental faculties.

Learning is a psychological process, not necessarily a logical one. Trying to frighten a student through threats of unsatisfactory reports or reprisals may seem logical, but is not effective psychologically. The effective instructor can organize teaching to fit the psychological needs of the student. If a situation seems overwhelming, the student feels unable to handle all of the factors involved, and a threat exists. So long as the student feels capable of coping with a situation, each new experience is viewed as a challenge.

A good instructor realizes that behaviour is directly influenced by the way a student perceives, and perception is affected by all of these factors. Therefore, it is important for the instructor to facilitate the learning process by avoiding any actions which may inhibit or prevent the attainment of teaching goals. Teaching is consistently effective only when those factors which influence perceptions are recognized and taken into account.

Insight

Insight involves the grouping of perceptions into meaningful wholes. Creating insight is one of the instructor's major responsibilities. To ensure that this does occur, it is essential to keep each student constantly receptive to new experiences and to help the student realize the way each piece relates to all other pieces of the total pattern of the task to be learned.

As an example, during straight-and-level flight in an airplane with a fixed-pitch propeller, the RPM will increase when the throttle is opened and decrease when it is closed. On the other hand, RPM changes can also result from changes in airplane pitch attitude without changes in power setting. Obviously, engine speed, power setting, airspeed, and airplane attitude are all related. True learning requires an understanding of how each of these factors may affect all of the others and, at the same time, knowledge of how a change in any one of them may affect all of the others. This mental relating and grouping of associated perceptions is called insight.

Insight will almost always occur eventually, whether or not instruction is provided. For this reason, it is possible for a person to become an electrician by trial and error, just as one may become a lawyer by reading law. Instruction, however, speeds this learning process by teaching the relationship of perceptions as they occur, thus promoting the development of the student's insight.

As perceptions increase in number and are assembled by the student into larger blocks of learning, they develop insight. As a result, learning becomes more meaningful and more permanent. Forgetting is less of a problem when there are more anchor points for tying insights together. It is a major responsibility of the instructor to organize demonstrations and explanations, and to direct practice, so that the student has better opportunities to understand the interrelationship of the many kinds of experiences that have been perceived. Pointing out the relationships as they occur, providing a secure and nonthreatening environment in which to learn, and helping the student acquire and maintain a favourable self-concept are key steps in fostering the development of insight.

Motivation

Motivation is probably the dominant force which governs the student's progress and ability to learn. Motivation may be negative or positive, tangible or intangible, subtle and difficult to identify, or it may be obvious.

Negative motivation may engender fear, and be perceived by the student as a threat. While negative motivation may be useful in certain situations, characteristically it is not as effective in promoting efficient learning as positive motivation.

Positive motivation is provided by the promise or achievement of rewards. These rewards may be personal or social; they may involve financial gain, satisfaction of the self-concept, or public recognition. Motivation which can be used to advantage by the instructor includes the desire for personal gain, the desire for personal comfort or security, the desire for group approval, and the achievement of a favourable self-image.

The desire for personal gain, either the acquisition of possessions or status, is a basic motivational factor for all human endeavour. An individual may be motivated to dig a ditch or to design a supersonic airplane solely by the desire for financial gain.

Students are like typical employees in wanting a tangible return for their efforts. For motivation to be effective, students must believe that their efforts will be suitably rewarded. These rewards must be constantly apparent to the student during instruction, whether they are to be financial, self-esteem, or public recognition.

Lessons often have objectives which are not obvious at first. Although these lessons will pay dividends during later instruction, the student may not appreciate this fact. It is important for the instructor to make the student aware of those applications which are not immediately apparent. Likewise, the devotion of too much time and effort to drill and practice on operations which do not directly contribute to competent performance should be avoided. The desire for personal comfort and security is a form of motivation which instructors often forget. All students want secure, pleasant conditions and a safe environment. If they recognize that what they are learning may promote these objectives, their attention is easier to attract and hold. Insecure and unpleasant training situations inhibit learning.

Everyone wants to avoid pain and injury. Students normally are eager to learn operations or procedures which help prevent injury or loss of life. This is especially true when the student knows that the ability to make timely decisions, or to act correctly in an emergency, is based on sound principles.

The attractive features of the activity to be learned also can be a strong motivational factor. Students are anxious to learn skills which may be used to their advantage. If they understand that each task will be useful in preparing for future activities, they will be more willing to pursue it.

Another strong motivating force is group approval. Every person wants the approval of peers and superiors. Interest can be stimulated and maintained by building on this natural desire. Most students enjoy the feeling of belonging to a group and are interested in accomplishment which will give them prestige among their fellow students. Every person seeks to establish a favourable self-image. In certain instances, this self-image may be submerged in feelings of insecurity or despondency. Fortunately, most people engaged in a task believe that success is possible under the right combination of circumstances and good fortune. This belief can be a powerful motivating force for students. An instructor can effectively foster this motivation by the introduction of perceptions which are solidly based on previously learned factual information that is easily recognized by the student. Each additional block of learning should help formulate insight which contributes to the ultimate training goals. This promotes student confidence in the overall training program and, at the same time, helps the student develop a favourable self-image. As this confirmation progresses and confidence increases, advances will be more rapid and motivation will be strengthened.

Positive motivation is essential to true learning. Negative motivation in the form of reproofs or threats should be avoided with all but the most overconfident and impulsive students. Slumps in learning are often due to declining motivation. Motivation does not remain at a uniformly high level. It may be affected by outside influences, such as physical or mental disturbances or inadequate instruction. The instructor should strive to maintain motivation at the highest possible level. In addition, the instructor should be alert to detect and counter any lapses in motivation.

Levels of Learning

Levels of learning may be classified in any number of ways. Four basic levels have traditionally been included in aviation instructor training. The lowest level is the ability to repeat something which one has been taught, without understanding or being able to apply what has been learned. This is referred to as rote learning. Progressively higher levels of learning are understanding what has been taught, achieving the skill for application of what has been learned, and correlation of what has been learned with other things previously learned or subsequently encountered.

For example, a flight instructor may explain to a beginning student the procedure for entering a level, left turn. The procedure may include several steps such as: (1) visually clear the area, (2) add a slight amount of power to maintain airspeed, (3) apply aileron control pressure to the left, (4) add sufficient rudder pressure in the direction of the turn to avoid slipping and skidding, and (5) increase back pressure to maintain altitude. A student who can verbally repeat this instruction has learned the procedure by rote. This will not be very useful to the student if there is never an opportunity to make a turn in flight, or if the student has no knowledge of the function of airplane controls.

With proper instruction on the effect and use of the flight controls, and experience in controlling the airplane during straight-and-level flight, the student can consolidate these old and new perceptions into an insight on how to make a turn. At this point, the student has developed an understanding of the procedure for turning the airplane in flight. This understanding is basic to effective learning, but may not necessarily enable the student to make a correct turn on the first attempt.

When the student understands the procedure for entering a turn, has had turns demonstrated, and has practiced turn entries until consistency has been achieved, the student has developed the skill to apply what has been learned. This is a major level of learning, and one at which the instructor is too often willing to stop. Discontinuing instruction on turn entries at this point and directing subsequent instruction exclusively to other elements of piloting performance is characteristic of piecemeal instruction, which is usually inefficient. It violates the building block concept of instruction by failing to apply what has been learned to future learning tasks. The building block concept will be covered later in more detail.

The correlation level of learning, which should be the objective of aviation instruction, is that level at which the student becomes able to associate an element which has been learned with other segments or blocks of learning. The other segments may be items or skills previously learned, or new learning tasks to be undertaken in the future. The student who has achieved this level of learning in turn entries, for example, has developed the ability to correlate the elements of turn entries with the performance of chandelier and lazy eights.

Domains of Learning

Besides the four basic levels of learning, educational psychologists have developed several additional levels. These classifications consider what is to be learned. Is it knowledge only, a change in attitude, a physical skill, or a combination of knowledge and skill? One of the more useful categorizations of learning objectives includes three domains: cognitive domain (knowledge), affective domain (attitudes, beliefs, and values), and psychomotor domain (physical skills). Each of the domains has a hierarchy of educational objectives.

The listing of the hierarchy of objectives is often called a taxonomy. A taxonomy of educational objectives is a systematic classification scheme for sorting learning outcomes into the three broad categories (cognitive, affective, and psychomotor) and ranking the desired outcomes in a developmental hierarchy from least complex to most complex.

Learning Experiences

Who says learning only happens in a controlled environment? Here's how you can turn regular chores and everyday activities into learning experiences.

A child begins to learn right from the time he is in his mother's womb. Experts say that at this time the mother feelings and experiences are all transferred to the baby. A couple of generations ago the elders in the family used to emphasise on the importance of reading the scriptures and 'feel good' stories so that its impact is felt on the baby.

Learning continues from when the baby is born and first experiences the world. As the child grows he learns by experimenting. You may find a toddler beating a few objects. He is learning unconsciously (and rather noisily) the different sounds each item makes. If we as parents make a conscious effort to provide different experiences to our child, he becomes a keen learner - learning from observation and experience - a skill he will benefit from throughout his life. Here are a few tips to make day-to-day activities a true learning experience for your children.

Distraction

Distraction is the diversion of attention of an individual or group from the chosen object of attention onto the source of distraction. Distraction is caused by one of the following: lack of ability to pay attention; lack of interest in the object of attention; greater interest in something other than the object of attention; or the great intensity, novelty or attractiveness of something other than the object of attention. Distractions come from both external sources (physical stimuli through the five senses), or internal sources (thought, emotion, fantasies, physical urges). Divided attention, as in multi-tasking could also be considered as distraction in situations requiring full attention on a single object (e.g. sports, academic tests, performance).

Distraction is a major cause of procrastination, though it is possible to be diligent and still diverted from what is valuable. According to philosopher Damon Young, distraction is chiefly an inability to identify, attend to or attain what is valuable, even when we are hard working or content. In works of fiction, distraction is often used as a source of comedy, whether the amusement comes from the gullibility of those distracted or the strangeness of whatever is utilized to create the distraction.

Division of Attention

Ten men were asked to listen to bursts of noise which were presented to one ear, and which might or might not contain a tone. The other ear received 6 digit numbers simultaneously. The listeners reported their degree of confidence that a tone was present; in one condition they ignored the numbers and in another condition they had to report them as well as their judgement about the tone. In the latter condition they reported the tone with confidence slightly less often when it was present, but also reported it more often when it was in fact absent. Analysis of the results, by a model which supposes the brain to detect signals by a statistical decision, shows that one parameter, β, is unchanged by division of attention. This parameter measures the subjective probabilities and values associated with signal as opposed to nonsignal. Another parameter, changes when attention is divided. This quantity measures the strength of the signal relative to the random variation within the system. It is concluded that diversion of attention away from a stimulus produces an effect resembling a reduction in the intensity of the stimulus. The ignored event is therefore not blocked altogether and under suitable conditions may nevertheless produce a response from an observer.

Learning Environment

"Learners in supportive environments have high levels of self efficacy and self-motivation and use learning as a primary transformative force" (Bereiter & Scardamalia, 1989).

To be effective, instructional multimedia should address the unique sources for learning differences that influence success. More specifically, it should emulate the instructor's experienced, intuitive ability to recognize and respond to how individuals learn differently and creatively foster interest, value, and more successful, independent learning. (Martinez, 1999).

An efficient way to accomplish this challenging task is to determine common learning-difference profiles and match individualized solutions to audiences differentiated by these profiles. This is actually simpler than it seems. Research helps us broadly describe four learning orientation profiles. Below are descriptions for mass customized learning environments that fit each of the learning orientations:

Transforming Learners prefer loosely structured, flexible mentoring environments that promote challenging goals, discovery, strategies, problem solving, and self-managed learning.

Performing Learners prefer semi-structured environments that stimulate personal value and provide details, tasks, processes, and creative interaction (hands-on) not exploration and great effort.

Conforming Learners prefer simple, safe, low-learner control, structured environments that help learners achieve comfortable, low-risk learning goals in a linear fashion.

These descriptions support the broad variability in learning from a whole-person perspective, not simply in cognitive terms. They consider how emotions and intentions influence learning and thinking processes. These are powerful influences that guide how successfully individuals intend to learn. A closely matched learning environment will clearly have a positive impact on the accessibility, affordability, and quality challenges that now confront global education and training.

Teacher and Teaching

Printer-friendly version of Section

Educational psychology continues to provide a major basis for the initial education of teachers, particularly in management of learning and behaviour, but also on curriculum design, with special attention given to the needs of individual children. Increasingly, educational psychology is also contributing to student teachers' understanding of the school as a system and the importance of this wider perspective for optimizing their performance; to their professional development by helping them analyse their own practice, beliefs, and attitudes and, once they begin the practice of teaching, to their continuing professional development based on experience in schools—particularly in areas such as special needs and disability. The impact of information technology and the increasing development of inclusive education provide particular challenges.

Significance of Educational Psychology to the Teacher

Over the years, educational psychology has been a part of teacher preparation, moving from a centerpiece in many programs, through periods when it was deemed irrelevant by some, to current concerns about its role in the reforming of teacher education and teaching. Today, psychological knowledge is used to ground reforms in teaching and schooling, particularly the call for teaching for understanding. Current standards for teacher certifications and licensure and suggestions for reform in teacher education assume that teachers will have a deep and generative understanding of learning, development, motivation, and individual differences. This article explores several themes that recur in the writing on reforms and teacher standards: the need to place learning at the centre of teaching, the call for integrated studies, and the value of collaboration with the public schools. These themes have both positive and negative implications for the role of educational psychology in teacher education.

For years, I have been interested in the role of educational psychology in teacher education (Woolfolk, 1989, 1993, 1994; Woolfolk Hoy, 1996a, 1996b, 1996c, 1996d, 1997a, 1997b, 1998a, 1998b, in press; Woolfolk Hoy & Murphy, 2001; Woolfolk Hoy & Tschannen-Moran, 1999). Discussions with colleagues across the country suggest that many share this concern. The overarching goal of this article is to examine the past and present status of educational psychology in the preparation of teachers. I focus on three themes that recur in the writing on teacher standards and reforms—themes that have implications for *what* about educational psychology teachers should learn and *how* that learning should take place. The themes are: (a) the centrality of student learning in teaching, (b) the call for integrated studies, and (c) the value of collaboration with the public schools.

This examination begins with a brief glance at the history of educational psychology in teacher education, then moves to consider how the content and focus of educational psychology have changed over the years as both teacher education faculty and students demanded greater relevance, application, and utility from the study of educational psychology.

Next, I look to the future by analyzing selected perspectives on standards and reforms in teaching and teacher preparation—most written by educators and policymakers outside educational psychology. What messages do these views of the future hold for our field? In many of these reform agendas are affirmations of the importance for teaching and teacher education of topics historically studied by educational psychologists, such as learning, development, motivation, and individual differences.

Although few teacher educators or policymakers over the years have questioned the value of psychological knowledge, there is less agreement about what exactly should be learned or how the learning should take place.

The third part of this article focuses on the three reform themes listed earlier. The first theme, student learning as the centre of teaching, has implications for what educational psychology should be taught. The last two themes, integrated studies and collaboration with the schools, are related to how the learning of educational psychology might take place. I suggest a few opportunities and dangers in embracing these reforms and then conclude by describing challenges for educational psychology in teacher education.

Educational Psychology for Teachers: Reforming Our Courses, Rethinking Our Roles

The Educational Psychology Division (Division 15) of the American Psychological Association created a committee to examine the teaching of educational psychology in the broader context of teacher education reform. The committee recommends that educational psychologists who participate in teacher education should help prospective teachers develop contemporary psychological perspectives. To select content and pedagogy that support this goal, educational psychology teachers should consider both recent conceptualizations of teaching and teachers' knowledge as complex phenomena and current assumptions about complex learning. Educational psychologists should also think about relationships with other teacher educators, the preparation and support of educational psychology teachers, and research and development about teaching educational psychology.

Becoming a K-12 teacher usually involves enrolment in a college or university program that culminates in teacher certification. Within the majority of these programs, there is a formal requirement for coursework about ideas that educational psychologists claim as their domain, such as learning and development, individual differences, instruction, motivation, and measurement. Such courses historically have been offered early in students' programs, and sometimes are considered (and even named) "foundations" for later study of teaching.

Educational psychology foundations courses were developed in the early part of this century to help upgrade the status of teacher education —to improve the scholarship and rigor of professional programs by posing a scientific basis for further study (L. Shulman, 1990). However, criticisms of the Requests for reprints should be sent to Linda Anderson, 116G Erickson Hall, Michigan State University, East Lansing, MI 48824, foundational metaphor and courses based upon it are now being raised by educational psychologists (Berliner, 1992; Peterson, Dickson, & Clark, 1990; L. Shulman, 1990) and other teacher educators (Doyle, 1990 a). Similar criticisms of foundational approaches to professional education are also heard in other fields (Hoshmand & Polkinghorne, 1992; Schon, 1983).

Unit-II

Human Growth and Development

Human Growth and Development is planned to acquaint you with developmental concepts in psychology and to give you an understanding of the basic dynamics, which underlie human behaviour at various stages in the lifespan. You will have the opportunity to study human development from conception through childhood. Course content will include important theoretical models of human development and such specific topics as genetics, learning, intelligence, socialization, personality, sex-role identification, language acquisition, and moral development.

You will be investigating these processes in relation to biological, psychological, socioeconomic and cultural factors. Your performance will be evaluated primarily by tests and the completion of two term projects. However, other criteria, such as written and oral reports, class participation and attendance, will be used as deemed appropriate by the professor.

Interaction of Nature and Nature

The nature-nurture debate has long been a topic of interest among psychologists. However, it can safely be said that choosing one side or the other in such a debate is an incorrect way to arrive at any logical conclusion; "Individual development is always the result of the interaction of nature and nurture" (Pinel, 2007, p.31). We are all different in complex ways; and it is not possible to quantify either the genetic or experiential components which produce a behaviour. When studying the development of two individuals, it is feasible to assume that genetics play a more substantial role in their development than experience, if the subjects are selected for their genetic similarities. However, when the subjects are unrelated, the contributions of genetics cannot be considered.

As an example of individual differences; a large group of 45 year old men are racing bicycles along a twenty mile route. They stay closely together for most of the journey, but toward the end of the race, several have fallen way behind. They all finish the race, but there is a 45 minute gap between the first and last competitors. Although they have all been riding the same brand of bicycle, the differences in performance can be attributed to their levels of fitness, and not the quality of the bicycle.

Nature and nurture cannot be used to measure individual differences, however, the interaction of both does account for individual development.

Concept, Distinction between Growth, Development and Maturation

The long period of development leading up to a modern human's adulthood arose relatively late in our evolutionary history, according to an analysis of growth patterns in fossil teeth in today's issue of the journal *Nature*.

The article was written by Christopher Dean of University College, London, and colleagues including Alan Walker, distinguished professor of anthropology and biology at Penn State.

"One of the things that sets modern humans apart from the living great apes is our long period of growth and development," Dean explains. "While humans take a good 18 to 20 years to grow up, other primate species like chimpanzees and gorillas take just 11 or 12 years."

A supporting article, written by Jacopo Moggi-Cecchi of the University of Florence in Italy, is included in the "News and Views" section of the journal. The research was designed to determine when the prolonged growth period we have today arose during our long evolutionary history.

"Dental development is a good measure of overall growth and development," says Walker, who pioneered the study of living primates as a basis for the analysis of fossils and was one of the first to use scanning electron microscope studies of fossil teeth.

Walker adds, "Teeth grow in an incremental manner like trees or shells, preserving a record of their growth with daily marks along the prisms that make up the enamel."

By making thin sections of modern and fossil teeth, the researchers were able to count the daily incremental markings within the enamel of humans, apes, and fossil "hominin" species in the human lineage in order to calculate and compare their rates of enamel formation.

"Of the 13 fossil tooth fragments we studied — both those attributed to the earliest australopith hominins that lived roughly between 4 and 1 million years ago, and those of the earliest members of our own Homo genus that lived about 1.5 million years ago — none showed the slower pattern of modern human enamel growth," says Walker, who in 1984 was a key member of the team that discovered a juvenile skeleton in Kenya from one of the earliest species in the Homo genus, Homo erectus. "We found that the first dental evidence for a modern human-like growth period appears much more recently, in a Neanderthal fossil that lived about 120,000 years ago."

The results are surprising because researchers had expected that Homo erectus — the first fossil human ancestor to show a suite of modern human-like characteristics including body proportions, body weight, and small teeth and jaws — would show evidence of a modern human-like growth period.

However, because the brain in Homo erectus was still not as large as a modern human's and because a long growth period is linked with the time needed to grow and learn to use a large brain, the researchers say these findings are compatible with predictions that could be made on the basis of brain size alone.

As part of their research, the scientists used the incremental growth markings to calculate the formation times of individual teeth as a clue in the solution to another mystery about the age at death of the Homo erectus fossil found in Kenya.

"Using these tooth-formation times, we can speculate about the age at which key teeth emerged into the mouth in Homo erectus," Dean explains. "It seems likely that the first permanent molar tooth, which erupts at around 6 years in modern humans and about 3.5 years in apes, erupted between 4 and 4.5 years in Homo erectus. Previously, most people accepted this boy was close to 11 or 12 years of age, but now it seems more likely he was closer to 8 years of age, which is a surprise because he was already 5 feet 3 inches tall."

"It seems our prolonged period of growth and development may be a more recent evolutionary acquisition that arose in step with our comparatively recent development of a larger, modern, human-sized brain," Walker says.

General Principles of Growth and Development: Characteristics, Dimensions of Development—Physical, Cognitive, Emotional, Social and Moral

We have learned that certain characteristics are typical of certain ages, but these are only guides and not set rules. Each child grows in his own way. One child may progress "slower" than another and still he is perfectly healthy and within the range of **development** appropriate for his age.

1. **Growth is a personal matter.** Each child grows in his own personal manner. He should be permitted to grow at his own rate. If you expect too much of him he does even less than he is able to do. If there is one thing a two year old child cannot do is to be four. Instead of comparing him to others and finding fault, accept him. Instead of nudging and pushing--nurture him.
2. **Growth comes from within.** We can encourage or we can hinder but the energy and the drive force that pushes a child to grow, is carried inside him. He desperately wants to grow and has the power within

to do it. Our job is to clear the track, guide him with loving acceptance and then relax and enjoy!

3. **Growth is gradual and orderly but uneven.** A child is gradually and continually moving toward maturity. We cannot and must not hurry him. Before he can run he must walk, before he can share, he must fully possess. He can never truly be an adult if he was not first fully a child. His **growth** may be likened to a spiral, bursting forward at a dizzying rate of speed, reaching the top and then maybe falling back, gathering strength, building reserves to make the steep climb again and always moving forward.
4. **Growth has certain characteristics common at particular stages: Birth to two years: "Can I trust you?"** Most of us feel pretty secure with babies, it's the children that drive us wild! Infancy is often called the age of trust. The infant is completely dependent on others to provide his needs. If they are met, he learns to trust his environment. He needs tender loving care.

Talk to him, play with him, he's perfectly delightful--don't worry about spoiling. Research has shown that it's the child who hasn't gotten enough attention or gets attention only when the adult feels like giving it that displays what we have called "spoiled" behaviour. Encourage him to try things for himself when he is ready, but remember that he wants to grow, you don't need to push him!

The two year old: "Will you let me be me?" The two year old typically is full of "no" and noise.

He's curious, which is fortunate because he has a lot to learn. He's very possessive which makes him rather a poor playmate. Forcing him to share is useless because forced sharing is not sharing at all. He snatches and grabs, pushes, slaps, hits, pinches, bites and resorts to any other available under-hand method of getting his own way. This means he needs supervision when he is playing with others, and one child at a time is about all he can handle. He's changeable. He may scream for a cracker and not eat it when you give it to him; he may clamour for a toy and indifferently toss it aside when he gets it; he is all "me do" one minute and "you do" the next. Making a choice is agony for him and he can dawdle forever. He needs the security of limits but he needs freedom, too. He must have an opportunity to develop his will and not always expect defeat.

The three year old: "Will you notice me?" The three year old is fairly peaceful. He generally tries to please, he can accept suggestions much better than the two year old, and he can make choices. The three year old is much more "civilized" than the two year old. He likes approval and will seek adult attention and sympathy. The ability to share and take turns appears. He plays well with one or two children, and even when conflicts occur he is often able to handle them without adult help. He still enjoys solitary play a great deal of the time. He is boastful. He can show extreme jealousy of a new baby and often reverts to baby behaviour when tired. He is beginning to be imaginative and loves to talk.

What Are the Big Five Dimensions of Personality?

Personality researchers have proposed that there are five basic dimensions of personality. Evidence of this theory has been growing over the past 50 years, beginning with the research of D. W. Fiske (1949) and later expanded upon by other researchers including Norman (1967), Smith (1967), Goldberg (1981), and McCrae & Costa (1987).

The "big five" are broad categories of personality traits. While there is a significant body of literature supporting this five-factor model of personality, researchers don't always agree the exact labels of each dimension. However, these five categories are usually described as follows:

1. **Extraversion:** This trait includes characteristics such as excitability, sociability, talkativeness, assertiveness, and high amounts of emotional expressiveness.
2. **Agreeableness:** This personality dimension includes attributes such as trust, altruism, kindness, affection, and other prosocial behaviours.
3. **Conscientiousness:** Common features of this dimension include high levels of thoughtfulness, with good impulse control and goal-directed behaviours.

Those high in conscientiousness tend to be organized and mindful of details.

4. **Neuroticism:** Individuals high in this trait tend to experience emotional instability, anxiety, moodiness, irritability, and sadness.
5. **Openness:** This trait features characteristics such as imagination and insight, and those high in this trait also tend to have a broad range of interests.

These dimensions represent broad areas of personality. Research has demonstrated that these groupings of characteristics tend to occur together in many people. For example, individuals who are sociable tend to be talkative. However, these traits do not always occur together. Personality is a complex and varied and each person may display behaviours across several of these dimensions.

Physical, Cognitive and Social-Emotional Human Development

The three areas of human development are physical, cognitive and social-emotional. These areas are different in many ways, but they also influence one another.

Physical development is characterized by patterns of physical growth and maturation. Other forms of physical development occurs in the genetic basis for some human characteristics and abilities, neurological (brain) development, the acquisition of motor skills. Physical developments also manifest themselves in the form of healthy and unhealthy behaviours. Cognitive development is associated with the changes in a person's reasoning. Cognitive developments are also reflected by a change in language. Developments of the cognitive sort also refer to memory, and concepts. An example of this is how a child's answers to a simple question may be very simple and an adult's answers are more complex, and use stronger vocabulary.

Social-emotional developments relate to the changes that occur in a person's feelings, ability to handle feelings and situations, and moral ideas. These developments also occur in relation to a person's social relationships. An increase or decrease in self confidence is a direct example of a social-emotional development.

It may appear that all of these areas are separate, but they are extremely closely related. For example "physical development (e.g., neurological growth) allows cognitive advancements to take place, and increases in the ability to look at situations from multiple perspectives (a cognitive ability) make possible more effective social relationships" (McDevitt & Ormrod, 2004, p. 6).

Imagine Johnny is a five-year-old boy attending his first year of school. Johnny will be changing and growing a lot in his first year of school. Physically he will be growing and getting taller. His motor schools will improve and he will be able to use his hands much better. Emotionally he will be learning how to interact in a controlled environment. He will be learning social skills such as sharing, and working together. He will also learn how to deal with emotions in group settings. Cognitively he will begin processing more information and learning the rules of the classroom environment. Johnny will be learning rights and wrongs and how to make decisions based on them.

As Johnny changes, this will cause an impact on his behaviour in the classroom. Johnny will be growing and may be bigger or smaller than most kids. This may cause Johnny to be shy or it may cause him to be more confident. Johnny may struggle with the emotions of dealing with many other children and this may cause him to act out or become timid. There are many possibilities that can occur in a school setting and it is important for a teacher to be aware of the different areas of development in order to nurture the student correctly.

Emotional Development

Ainsworth defines attachment as "an affectional tie that one person forms to another specific person, binding them together in space, and enduring over time ... [It] is discriminating and specific." It is not present at birth, but is developed. In a word, attachment means love. Attachment behaviours such as crying, smiling, physical contact, and vocalizing are the means by which attachment is forged but are not to be equated with the more abstract, underlying construct of attachment. Attachment theory is strongly based on ethological notions. Thus, attachment is seen as serving a biological function, that is, the protection of infants by ensuring their proximity to (attached) adults. The common goal of attached individuals is proximity. Bowlby was influenced by Freud's psychoanalytic theory of development, but argues that there is a primary biological need to become attached to at least one adult, whereas Freud argued that love for a mother was secondary to her satisfaction of an infant's hunger.

Intellectual Development

For Piaget, intelligence is defined as the ability to adapt to the environment, an ability that depends upon physical and psychological (cognitive) organization. The adaptation process has two complementary components, assimilation and accommodation. Assimilation refers to the tendency to process new information, sometimes with distortion, in terms of existing cognitive structures. Accommodation refers to the opposite process, that is, the modification of existing cognitive structures in response to new information. An individual strives for equilibrium between assimilation and accommodation, with thought being neither unrealistic (excessive assimilation) nor excessively realistic and hence disorganized (excessive accommodation).

For Piaget, cognition gradually becomes abstracted from perception over the course of 12 years. Infants begin cognitive exploration by actively perceiving and reflexively manipulating objects, giving the name sensorimotor period to the first phase of intellectual development. Perception is a key form of early cognitive activity, especially with newborns. The newborn infant can see, hear, smell, taste, and feel much better than previously thought, though sensitivity in these areas improves throughout the first year of life. Between the ages of 18 and 24 months, infants become capable of symbolic representation, occasionally solving problems just by thinking about them. The major accomplishment of the sensorimotor period is object permanence, the realization that objects continue to exist even when not observable. During the next 5 years, sometimes termed the preoperational period, children work on concrete operations such as classifying objects into categories, arranging things in serial order, figuring out causes and effects, or understanding a one-to-one correspondence of numbers to objects counted. They also eventually manipulate reality enough to overcome perceptual illusions such as that an amount of water changes when it is poured from a short wide glass into a tall narrow glass. From 7 to 11 years, children further consolidate their concrete mental operations. At about 12 years, many adolescents enter the final stage of intellectual development: formal operations. They become capable of abstract, logical thought. They understand reality as a subset of possible worlds, and are able to form multiple, systematic hypotheses, involving all possible combinations of relevant variables, in order to explain things. Many quarrel with Piaget's age assessments of children, but most people accept his sequence of stages as useful for classifying children.

Moral Development

L. Kohl-berg's work on moral development spans the chasm between intellectual and emotional development. He studied reasoning about hypothetical moral dilemmas, such as whether a person should steal an unaffordable drug in order to save someone's life. He classified such reasoning in six stages. At birth children are considered to be premoral. By the age of 7, most children are in stage 1, chiefly characterized by the belief that people should act in certain ways in order to avoid physical or other punishment. In 2 or 3 years, children reason primarily in terms of doing things for rewards; this is stage 2. Stage 3 involves reasoning focused less on rewards than on maintaining the approval of others. Stage 4 involves reasoning that unquestioningly accepts conventional rules. Actions are judged by a rigid set of regulations, religious, legal, or both. Most individuals do not develop past this point. A few, however, do reach postconventional moral reasoning, stage 5. These individuals think in terms of moral principles. Rarely, a step higher to stage 6 is reached, governed by original abstract moral principles such as articulaton of the golden rule. Kohlberg argued that moral development is progressive, without regression to earlier stages.

Social and Emotional Development

Developmental psychologists who are interested in social development examine how individuals develop social and emotional competencies. For example, they study how children form friendships, how they understand and deal with emotions, and how identity develops. Research in this area may involve study of the relationship between cognition or cognitive development and social behaviour.

Toddler

Intelligence is demonstrated through the use of symbols, language use matures, and memory and imagination are developed. Thinking is done in a nonlogical, nonreversible manner. Egocentric thinking predominates. Socially, toddlers are little people attempting to become independent at this stage, which they are commonly called the " terrible twos". They walk, talk, use the toilet, and get food for themselves. Self-control begins to develop. If taking the initiative to explore, experiment, risk mistakes in trying new things, and test their limits is encouraged by the caretaker(s) the child will become autonomous, self-reliant, and confident. If the caretaker is overprotective or disapproving of independent actions, the toddler may begin to doubt their abilities and feel ashamed for the desire for independence. The child's autonomic development will be inhibited, and be less prepared to successfully deal with the world in the future.

Phases of Development and Developmental Tasks—Infancy, Childhood and Adolescence

Early Childhood

When children attend preschool, they broaden their social horizons and become more engaged with those around them. Impulses are channelled into fantasies, which leaves the task of the caretaker to balance eagerness for pursuing adventure, creativity and self expression with the development of responsibility. If caretakers are properly encouraging and consistently disciplinary, children are more likely to develop positive self-esteem while becoming more responsible, and will follow through on assigned activities. If not allowed to decide which activities to perform, children may begin to feel guilt upon contemplating taking initiative. This negative association with independence will lead them to let others make decisions in place of them.

Childhood

In middle childhood, intelligence is demonstrated through logical and systematic manipulation of symbols related to concrete objects. Operational thinking develops, which means actions are reversible, and egocentric thought diminishes.

Children go through the transition from the world at home to that of school and peers. Children learn to make things, use tools, and acquire the skills to be a worker and a potential provider. Children can now receive feedback from outsiders about their accomplishments. If children can discover pleasure in intellectual stimulation, being productive, seeking success, they will develop a sense of competence. If they are not successful or cannot discover pleasure in the process, they may develop a sense of inferiority and feelings of inadequacy that may haunt them throughout life. This is when children think of them selves as industrious or as inferior

Adolescence

Adolescence is the period of life between the onset of puberty and the full commitment to an adult social role, such as worker, parent, and/or citizen. It is the period known for the formation of personal and social identity and the discovery of moral purpose. Intelligence is demonstrated through the logical use of symbols related to abstract concepts and formal reasoning. A return to egocentric thought often occurs early in the period. Only 35% develop the capacity to reason formally during adolescence or adulthood. The adolescent asks "Who am I? Who do I want to be?" Like toddlers, adolescents must explore, test limits, become autonomous, and commit to an identity, or sense of self. Different roles, behaviours and ideologies must be tried out to select an identity. Role confusion and inability to choose vocation can result from a failure to achieve a sense of identity.

Early Adulthood

The person must learn how to form intimate relationships, both in friendship and love. The development of this skill relies on the resolution of other stages. It may be hard to establish intimacy if one has not developed trust or a sense of identity. If this skill is not learned the alternative is alienation, isolation, a fear of commitment, and the inability to depend on others. A related framework for studying this part of the life span is that of Emerging adulthood, introduced in 2000 by Jeffrey Arnett. Scholars of emerging adulthood are interested not only in relationship development (focusing on the role of dating in helping individuals settle on a long-term spouse/partner), but also the development of sociopolitical views and occupational choice.

Middle Age

Middle adulthood generally refers to the period between ages 40 to 65. During this period, the middle-aged experience a conflict between generativity and stagnation. They may either feel a sense of contributing to the next generation and their community or a sense of purposelessness. Physically, the middle-aged experience a decline in muscular strength, reaction time, sensory keenness, and cardiac output. Also, women experience menopause and a sharp drop in the hormone estrogen. Men do not have an equivalent to menopause, but they do experience a decline in sperm count and speed of ejaculation and erection. Most men and women remain capable of sexual satisfaction after middle age.

Old Age

This stage generally refers to those over 75 years. During old age, people experience a conflict between integrity vs. despair. When reflecting on their life, they either feel a sense of accomplishment or failure. Physically, older people experience a decline in muscular strength, reaction time, stamina, hearing, distance perception, and the sense of smell. They also are more susceptible to severe diseases such as cancer and pneumonia due to a weakened immune system. Mental disintegration may also occur, leading to Dementia or Alzheimer's Disease. However, partially due to a lifetime's accumulation of antibodies, the elderly are less likely to suffer from common diseases such as the cold or flu. Whether or not intellectual powers increase or decrease with age remains controversial. Longitudinal studies have suggested that intellect declines, while cross-sectional studies suggest that intellect is stable. It is generally believed that crystallized intelligence increases up to old age, while fluid intelligence decreases with age.

Developmental Tasks

A developmental task is one that arises predictably and consistently at or about a certain period in the life of the individual (Havighurst, 1948, 1953). The concept of developmental tasks assumes that human development in modern societies is characterized by a long series of tasks that individuals have to learn throughout their lives. Some of these tasks are located in childhood and adolescence, whereas others arise during adulthood and old age. Successful achievement of a certain task is expected to lead to happiness and to success with later tasks, while failure may result in unhappiness in the individual, disapproval by the society, and difficulty with later tasks.

Developmental tasks arise from three different sources (Havighurst, 1948, 1953). First, some are mainly based on physical maturation (e.g., learning to walk). Another source of developmental tasks relates to sociostructural and cultural forces. Such influences are based on, for instance, laws (e.g., minimum age for marriage) and culturally shared expectations of development (e.g., age norms; Neugarten, Moore, and Lowe, 1965), determining the age range in which specific developmental tasks have to be mastered. The third source of developmental tasks involves personal values and aspirations. These personal factors result from the interaction between ontogenetic and environmental factors, and play an active role in the emergence of specific developmental tasks (e.g., choosing a certain occupational pathway).

Childhood and Adolescence

Early childhood is characterized by basic tasks such as learning to walk, to take solid food, and to control the elimination of body wastes. In addition, young children have to achieve more complex cognitive and social tasks, such as learning to talk, to form simple concepts of reality, and to relate emotionally to other people. In middle childhood, developmental tasks relate to the expansion of the individual's world outside of the home (e.g., getting along with age mates, learning skills for culturally valued games) and to the mental thrust into the world of adult concepts and communication (e.g., skills in writing, reading, and calculating). Achieving adolescent developmental tasks requires a person to develop personal independence and a philosophy of life. Adolescents are confronted, for example, with learning to achieve new forms of intimate relationships, preparing for an occupation, achieving emotional independence of parents, and developing a mature set of values and ethical principals. The peer group plays a major role in facilitating the achievement of adolescents' developmental tasks by providing a context in which some of these tasks can be accomplished.

Adulthood and Old Age

The concept of developmental tasks describes development as a lifelong process. Thus, it is also an early and significant contributor to the emerging field of lifelong human development (e.g., life-span psychology and life-course sociology; Setterstery, 1999).

In young adulthood, developmental tasks are mainly located in family, work, and social life. Family-related developmental tasks are described as finding a mate, learning to live with a marriage partner, having and rearing children, and managing the family home. A developmental task that takes an enormous amount of time of young adults relates to the achievement of an occupational career. Family and work-related tasks may represent a potential conflict, given that individuals' time and energy are limited resources. Thus, young adults may postpone one task in order to secure the achievement of another. With respect to their social life, young adults are also confronted with establishing new friendships outside of the marriage and assuming responsibility in the larger community.

During midlife, people reach the peak of their control over the environment around them and their personal development. In addition, social responsibilities are maximized. Midlife is also a period during which people confront the onset of physiological changes (Lachman, 2001). Developmental tasks during midlife relate to, for example, achieving adult responsibilities, maintaining a standard of living, assisting children with the transition into adulthood, and adjusting to the physiological changes of middle age (e.g., menopause). Old age has often been characterized as a period of loss and decline. However, development in any period of life consists of both gains and losses, although the gain-loss ratio becomes increasingly negative with advancing age (Heckhausen, Dixon, and Baltes, 1989; Baltes, 1987). A central developmental task that characterizes the transition into old age is adjustment to retirement. The period after retirement has to be filled with new projects, but is characterized by few valid cultural guidelines. Adaptation to retirement involves both potential gains (e.g., self-actualization) and losses (e.g., loss of self-esteem). The achievement of this task may be obstructed by the management of another task, living on a reduced income after retirement. In addition, older adults are generally challenged to create a positive sense of their lives as a whole. The feeling that life has had order and meaning results in happiness (cf. ego-integrity; Erikson, 1986). Older adults also have to adjust to decreasing physical strength and health. The prevalence of chronic and acute diseases increases in old age. Thus, older adults may be confronted with life situations that are characterized by not being in perfect health, serious illness, and dependency on other people. Moreover, older adults may become caregivers to their spouses (e.g., Schulz and Beach, 1999). Some older adults have to adjust to the death of their spouses. This task arises more frequently for women than for man. After they have lived with a spouse for many decades, widowhood may force older people to adjust to loneliness, moving to a smaller place, and learning about business matters.

Unit-III

Cognitive Development

Probably the most cited theory in the cognitive development in children is Jean Piaget (1896-1980). As with all stage theories, *Piaget's Theory of Cognitive Development* maintains that children go through specific stages as their intellect and ability to see relationships matures. These stages are completed in a fixed order with all children, even those in other countries. The age range, however can vary from child to child.

Sensorimotor Stage: This stage occurs between the ages of birth and two years of age, as infants begin to understand the information entering their sense and their ability to interact with the world. During this stage, the child learns to manipulate objects although they fail to understand the permanency of these objects if they are not within their current sensory perception. In other words, once an object is removed from the child's view, he or she is unable to understand that the object still exists.

The major achievement during this stage is that of ***Object Permanency***, or the ability to understand that these objects do in fact continue to exist. This includes his ability to understand that when mom leaves the room, she will eventually return, resulting in an increased sense of safety and security. Object Permanency occurs during the end of this stage and represents the child's ability to maintain a mental image of the object (or person) without the actual perception.

Preoperational Stage: The second stage begins after Object Permanency is achieved and occurs between the ages of two to seven years of age. During this stage, the development of language occurs at a rapid pace. Children learn how to interact with their environment in a more complex manner through the use of words and images. This stage is marked by Egocentrism, or the child's belief that everyone sees the world the same way that she does. The fail to understand the differences in perception and believe that inanimate objects have the same perceptions they do, such as seeing things, feeling, hearing and their sense of touch. A second important factor in this stage is that of Conservation, which is the ability to understand that quantity does not change if the shape changes. In other words, if a short and wide glass of water is poured into a tall and thin glass. Children in this stage will perceive the taller glass as having more water due only because of it's height. This is due to the children's inability to understand *reversibility* and to focus on only one aspect of a stimulus (called ***centration***), such as height, as opposed to understanding other aspects, such as glass width.

Concrete Operations Stage: Occurring between ages 7 and about 12, the third stage of cognitive development is marked by a gradual decrease in centristic thought and the increased ability to focus on more than one aspect of a stimulus. They can understand the concept of grouping, knowing that a small dog and a large dog are still both dogs, or that pennies, quarters, and dollar bills are part of the bigger concept of money.

They can only apply this new understanding to concrete objects (those they have actually experienced). In other words, imagined objects or those they have not seen, heard, or touched, continue to remain somewhat mystical to these children, and abstract thinking has yet to develop.

Formal Operations Stage: In the final stage of cognitive development (from age 12 and beyond), children begin to develop a more abstract view of the world. They are able to apply reversibility and conservation to both real and imagined situations. They also develop an increased understanding of the world and the idea of cause and effect. By the teenage years, they are able to develop their own theories about the world. This stage is achieved by most children, although failure to do so has been associated with lower intelligence.

Cognitive Process

It has been observed since antiquity that language acquisition in human children fails to emerge unless the children are exposed to language. Thus, language acquisition is an example of an emergent behaviour. In this case, the individual is made up of a set of mechanisms 'expecting' such input from the social world.

In education, for instance, which has the explicit task in society of developing child cognition, choices are made regarding the environment and permitted action that lead to a formed experience. In social cognition, face perception in human babies emerges by the age of two months. This is in turn affected by the risk or cost of providing these, for instance, those associated with a playground or swimming pool or field trip. On the other hand, the macro-choices made by the teachers are extremely influential on the micro-choices made by children.

In a large systemic perspective, cognition is considered closely related to the social and human organization functioning and constrains. Managerial decision making processes can be erroneous in politics, economy and industry for the reason of different reciprocally dependent socio-cognitive factors. This domain became the field of interest of emergent socio-cognitive engineering.

Attention—Factors relating to Attention

Children (ages 5, 7, and 9 years) and young adults completed two visual attention tasks that required them to make a forced choice identification response to a target shape presented in the centre of a computer screen. In the first task (high correlation condition) each target was flanked with the same distracters on 80% of the trials (valid flanker), with the other flanker on 10% of the trials (invalid flanker) and alone on 10% of the trials. In the second task (low correlation condition), targets were paired with valid flankers on 48% of trials, invalid flankers on 40% of trials, and alone on 12% of trials. Degree of attention focus was varied by presenting a fixation point at the target location on 50% of the trials, and target flanker similarity was also varied. Reaction times and accuracy were measured in various conditions to assess the degree of learning associated with high probability stimulus pairings, and the extent to which the learning would transfer to the subsequent low correlation condition. Results suggest that children are more likely to focus attention with a fixation point than without, and may be less likely to mediate their response times with increasing task difficulty. Results are explained with reference to attention control deficit hypotheses related to cognitive development.

Kinds of Attention—Inattention, Distraction and Division of Attention

Predominantly Inattentive ADHD can go unnoticed because children with this type of ADHD do not display behaviour that is particularly disruptive. According to the *National Institute of Mental Health*, children with this type of ADHD rarely experience symptoms of impulsivity or hyperactivity. Often described as forgetful or sluggish, children experiencing symptoms of inattention need treatment just as much as those experiencing the more disrupting symptoms of hyperactivity and impulsivity.

How do you distinguish between normal childhood behaviour and the symptoms of ADHD? According to the *National Institute of Mental Health*, children with ADHD may also experience some of the following symptoms of inattention:

Children who are inattentive have a hard time keeping their minds on any one thing and may get bored with a task after only a few minutes. If they are doing something they really enjoy, they have no trouble paying attention. But focusing deliberate, conscious attention to organizing and completing a task or learning something new is difficult.

Homework is particularly hard for these children. They will forget to write down an assignment, or leave it at school. They will forget to bring a book home, or bring the wrong one. The homework, if finally finished, is full of errors and erasures. Homework is often accompanied by frustration for both parent and child.

Span of Attention

Length of the Span

Attention span varies with age, with older children capable of longer periods of attention than younger children. The type of activity is also an important consideration, as people are generally capable of a longer attention span when they are doing something that they find enjoyable or intrinsically motivating.

Estimates for the length of human attention span are highly variable and range from 3 to 5 minutes per year of age in young children, to a maximum of around 20 minutes in adults. Nevertheless, the average movie lasts approximately two hours, and most adults can follow the plot with only minimal lapses of attention.

Continuous attention span, or the amount of time a human can focus on an object without any lapse at all, is very brief and may be as short as 8 seconds. After this amount of time, it is likely that an individual's eyes will shift focus, or that a stray thought will briefly enter consciousness. Fortunately, these short lapses are only minimally distracting and do not tend to interfere with task performance.

Effects of Temperament

In an early study of attention span, the mothers of 232 pairs of twins were interviewed periodically about the similarities and differences in behaviour displayed by their twins during infancy and early childhood. The results showed that each of the behavioural variables (temper frequency, temper intensity, irritability, crying, and demanding attention) had a significant inverse relationship with attention span. In other words, the twin with longer attention span, who was better able to remain absorbed in a particular activity without distraction, was also the less temperamental twin.

Historical Differences

The attention span of humans is apparently much shorter than it used to be. Neil Postman discusses this in his book, *Amusing Ourselves to Death*. One of his examples is the Lincoln-

Douglas debates of 1858. These lasted for hours in front of a sustained audience, whereas modern debates do not approach that length.

The instant gratification made possible by modern technology appears to have had a detrimental effect on attention span. One study of 2600 children found that early exposure to television (around age two) is associated with later attention problems at age seven. Internet browsing may have a similar effect because it enables rapid viewing. Most internet users spend less than one minute on the average website. It may be wise for parents to limit television and internet use in children and encourage them to read books instead. A gradual progression to longer books could be an effective way to develop a healthy attention span.

Sensation

Sleep loss, excessive fatigue, stress and inattention constitute the social diseases of our century. Within the "24 hour society" people tend more and more to exchange sleep and serenity for gain or pleasure. This gradually leads to an excessive rate of sleep disorders, roughly 20% of the population suffer from one, at least mildly or temporarily, as well as to a boom of stress and anxiety related diseases. In addition, a significant percentage of severe traffic and industrial accidents seem to be caused by the involuntary human transition from wakefulness to sleep or by prolonged inattention.

SENSATION aims to explore a wide range of micro and nano sensor technologies, with the aim to achieve unobtrusive, cost-effective, real-time monitoring, detection and prediction of human physiological state in relation to wakefulness, fatigue and stress anytime, everywhere and for everybody.

Thus, the different states of human brain are analysed within Subproject 1. In Subproject 2, 17 micro sensors and 2 nano sensors are developed. They include brain monitoring, wearable, eye-related posture and motility and autonomic functions sensors; all wirelessly integrated through a body/local/wide area network. These sensors are combined into medical systems for medical diagnosis and treatment within

Subproject 3. They will be also integrated in a system for operator's hypovigilance detection and prediction, to be used in various industrial operations and environments within Subproject 4. The overall IP is coordinated by a series of cross-project activities within Subproject 5.

Perception

In philosophy, psychology, and the cognitive sciences, perception is the process of attaining awareness or understanding of sensory information. It is a task far more complex than was imagined in the 1950s and 1960s, when it was predicted that building perceiving machines would take about a decade, a goal which is still very far from fruition. The word comes from the Latin words *perceptio, percipio,* and means "receiving, collecting, action of taking possession, apprehension with the mind or senses."

Perception is one of the oldest fields in psychology. The oldest quantitative law in psychology is the Weber-Fechner law, which quantifies the relationship between the intensity of physical stimuli and their perceptual effects. The study of perception gave rise to the Gestalt school of psychology, with its emphasis on holistic approach.

What one perceives is a result of interplays between past experiences, including one's culture, and the interpretation of the perceived. If the percept does not have support in any of these perceptual bases it is unlikely to rise above perceptual threshold.

Factors relating to Perception, Perceptual Errors

Perception is one of the oldest and most fundamental disciplines within Psychology., dating back to at least the time of the ancient Greeks. The goal of perception research is to understand how stimuli from the world interact with our sensory systems, forming visual, auditory, tactile, olfactory, and gustatory representations of the world. Research in perception and psychophysics is directed at discovering the lawful relations between environmental events and subjective experience. This area spans a wide range of problems extending from the structure and function of the sense organs, through the processing of sensory information, to the nature of subjective experience and the methods by which an accurate description of these experiences is obtained. As such, an understanding of perception is critical for all areas within Psychology. The modern study of perception is highly integrative, combining cognitive, behavioural, computational, developmental, and neuroscientific approaches.

Cognitive Factors

Perception is the processing of applying stored knowledge to the sensory input and forming an interpretation. Once the image is sensed, the officer must decide whether it represents a gun or some other object based on what he knows and what he has learned through experience. When the sensory information is uncertain or ambiguous, as with low visibility, the cognitive factors grow in importance.

This is a problem-solving task that humans address by using innate cognitive strategies. In psychology they are called "heuristics," general rules of thumb, or "biases." The term "bias" is not meant in the negative sense of everyday language. In cognitive psychology, a "basis" is a reasoning strategy that aids in quickly arriving at a correct answer. In critical situations, it is dangerous to engage in the slow process of conscious reasoning. Instead, the human mind has evolved heuristics and biases to speed the interpretation and to make sense of a complex situation.

Here are some of the major cognitive heuristics and biases. It is important to remember that these are innate and "normal," in the sense that virtually all humans rely on them heavily. Further, they operate unconsciously, so that most people are unaware that their interpretations are affected by such operations.

1. *Experience creates expectation.* People become skilled at their jobs through learning and development of expectation. Beginners act is a "controlled" mode, where they must stop and consciously think about every decision. Their performance is slow and inefficient and

usually errorful. With learning, people switch to a fast and "automatic" mode where responses seem to occur without conscious thought or decision. Part of the shift occurs because the skilled person learns what to expect, and can act without the need conscious decision-making, such as recognizing objects.

While it is often said, "see is believing," it is equally true that "believing is seeing." Officers who have previously been in situations where a suspect was armed, for example, have more reason to believe that future suspects will be armed and are far more likely to expect to see a gun. However, the experience need not be firsthand. If the station house talk dwells in instances of suspects with weapons, officers shot by suspects, etc., this can also sway expectation in favour of interpreting indistinct objects as guns.

2. *The "availability heuristic" primes perception.* People must use information stored in memory to make decisions. In a critical situation, they will most likely use the first information that comes to mind. One factor that causes quick recall is that the information was recently acquired. In general, the most recently learned information is what most readily comes to mind, i.e. is most available in memory. Recently read or heard information is the most available and is likely to have the strongest influence on decision-making and on interpretation of low visibility objects.

   For an officer going out on patrol, the most available information may originate in the pre-patrol briefing. For example, the officers may be reminded to keep an eye out for a dangerous suspect of a specific description or that there have been reports of violent crimes an specific area. When the officer later must make a split-second decision, s/he draws on memory in order interpret the ambiguous visual information. S/he is especially likely to perceive a gun if the suspect fits the general description of the dangerous suspect or is located is the area where violent crimes occur.

3. *"Confirmation Bias" strengthens preconceived beliefs.* Confirmation bias refers to the tendency to seek information that supports and already held belief and to avoid or dismiss evidence that contradicts it. It is perhaps the most powerful cognitive bias, and has been found to be a source of error and accident across a wide spectrum of human activities.

   If an officer believes that a person is likely to be a suspect (he matches a description, is located in a high crime area, acting strangely, etc.) s/he will likely form an opinion that the person is potentially dangerous. Once this belief takes hold, the officer will look for evidence to support the belief and ignore, avoid, or rationalize evidence that contradicts it. When the person appears with an object in his hand, it will be interpreted as a gun. This conclusion confirms the initial belief that the suspect is dangerous.
4. *Payoffs affect decision-making.* A person who must decide under uncertain conditions, such as low visibility, faces the quandary that is depicted. S/he must decide whether a "signal" is present or whether there is only "noise." (The terms "signal" and "noise" arose from the "Signal Detection Theory," a mathematical analysis originally used as a model of radar operators-how did they decide whether there was an enemy plane on the screen or merely background noise.) For an officer who sees the object in the viewer's hand, the "signal" is a gun and the noise is an innocuous object.

Concept Formation: Nature and Types of Concepts—Piaget's Stages of Cognitive Development

Ayn Rand's Formulation

The first step in concept formation, called *differentiation,* is to isolate two or more things as belonging together, as *units* of the same class. Where many theories of concept formation hold that such isolation begins by noticing degrees of similarity, Objectivism holds that it starts by noticing degrees of differences. At the perceptual level, everything is different; however, somethings are more different from others. The difference between two tables, for instance, is less than the difference between a table and a chair. Because two tables are less different from one another when contrasted against a third object, we group them together as *units,* as members of a group of similar objects.

Ayn Rand defines similarity as: *the relationship between two or more existents which possess the same characteristic(s), but in different measure or degree.* Similarity is a matter of measurement. Going back to the table versus chair example, the difference between tables is a quantitative one-we can easily *stretch* one table into another, so we call them similar. The difference between tables and chairs, on the other hand, is qualitative, so we distinguish between these as belonging to another group. Of course, at a broader level, even the difference between tables and chairs is quantitative-with enough stretching and pulling one could turn a chair into a table as well. However, the point is that the table-to-table stretching is much less than the table-to-chair stretching, so we consider one quantitative and the other qualitative.

The second step of concept formation, *integration,* is based on a process Ayn Rand called *measurement omission.* In this step, we combine or integrate the units into a new, single mental unit by eliding the quantitative differences between the two units. We retain the characteristics of the units, but we elide the particular measurements-on the principle that these measurements must exist in some quantity, but may exist in any quantity. For example, when forming the concept *table* we retain the distinguishing characteristics-a flat, level surface and supports-but omit the particular measurements of those features.

Childhood Intelligence

Psychologists and other authorities are keenly interested in childhood intelligence. Intelligence is an inferred cognitive capacity that relates to a person's knowledge, adaptation, and ability to reason and act purposefully. Around the beginning of the twentieth century, Alfred Binet and Theophile Simon measured perception, memory, and vocabulary in children. These researchers divided a child's mental age, or level of intellectual attainment, by his or her chronological age, or actual age, to yield the child's intelligence quotient (IQ). Years later, the average IQ for a child was set at 100. Today, the two most famous IQ tests for children are the Stanford-Binet Intelligence Scale and the Wechsler Intelligence Scale for Children (WISC), both of which have been updated numerous times. Some psychologists indicate that the multifaceted nature of intelligence necessitates a distinction between basic intelligence (academic IQ) and applied intelligence (practical IQ). For instance, Howard Gardner proposed that children exhibit multiple intelligences, including musical ability, complex movement, and empathy. Similarly, Robert Sternberg proposed the triarchic theory of intelligence, which states that intelligence consists of three factors: information-processing skills, context, and experience. These three factors determine whether cognition or behaviour is intelligent.

An individual's intelligence, at least as measured by IQ tests, remains fairly constant throughout life. Yet considerable differences in IQ scores exist across a range of individuals. These individual differences are probably the result of some combination of genetics, home and educational environment, motivation, nutrition and health, socioeconomic status, and culture.

Critics repeatedly question the value of measuring intelligence, especially when the most commonly used testing instruments are inherently culture-specific. Critics point out that minorities score lower on IQ tests that are devised and standardized using white, middle-class subjects. These same minorities score higher on IQ tests devised and standardized using subjects from their own cultural background. Proponents of IQ tests suggest that it is possible to develop culture-fair (fair for all members in a culture) and culture-free (without cultural content) IQ tests, such as Raven's Progressive Matrices Test. This IQ test gauges the subject's ability to solve problems that are presented in unfamiliar designs. Proponents also claim that IQ scores effectively predict future academic performance—

what these tests were originally designed to measure. A great deal of uproar occurred in the 1970s in response to schools placing minorities into special education classes based on their IQ scores. These scores were obtained from culturally biased IQ tests. Today, IQ tests cannot be used as academic achievement or placement tests.

Piagets Theory of Cognitive Development

The **Theory of Cognitive Development**, one of the most historically influential theories was developed by Jean Piaget, a Swiss psychologist (1896–1980). His theory provided many central concepts in the field of developmental psychology and concerned the growth of intelligence, which for Piaget, meant the ability to more accurately represent the world and perform logical operations on representations of concepts grounded in the world. The theory concerns the emergence and acquisition of schemata—schemes of how one perceives the world—in "developmental stages", times when children are acquiring new ways of mentally representing information. The theory is considered "constructivist", meaning that, unlike nativist theories (which describe cognitive development as the unfolding of innate knowledge and abilities) or empiricist theories (which describe cognitive development as the gradual acquisition of knowledge through experience), it asserts that we construct our cognitive abilities through self-motivated action in the world. For his development of the theory, Piaget was awarded the Erasmus Prize. Piaget divided schemes that children use to understand the world through four main periods, roughly correlated with and becoming increasingly sophisticated with age:

- Sensorimotor period (years 0–2)
- Preoperational period (years 2–7)
- Concrete operational period (years 7–11)
- Formal operational period (years 11–adulthood)

Sensorimotor Period

According to Piaget, this child is in the *sensor-imotor period* and primarily explores the world with senses rather than through mental operations. Infants are born with a set of congenital reflexes, according to Piaget, in addition to a drive to explore their world. Their initial schemas are formed through differentiation of the congenital reflexes.

The ***sensorimotor period*** is the first of the four periods. According to Piaget, this stage marks the development of essential spatial abilities and understanding of the world in six sub-stages:

1. The first substage, known as *the reflex schema* stage, occurs from birth to six weeks and is associated primarily with the development of reflexes.
2. The second substage, *primary circular reaction phase*, occurs from six weeks to four months and is associated primarily with the development of habits.
3. The third substage, the *secondary circular reactions phase*, occurs from four to nine months and is associated primarily with the development of coordination between vision and prehension.
4. The fourth substage, called *the coordination of secondary circular reactions stage*, which occurs from nine to twelve months, is when Piaget (1954) thought that object permanence developed.
5. The fifth substage, *the tertiary circular reactions phase*, occurs from twelve to eighteen months and is associated primarily with the discovery of new means to meet goals.
6. The sixth substage, considered "beginnings of symbolic representation", is associated primarily with the beginnings of insight, or true creativity.

Preoperational Stage

The Preoperational stage is the second of four stages of cognitive development. By observing sequences of play, Piaget was able to demonstrate that towards the end of the second year a qualitatively new kind of psychological functioning occurs.

(Pre) Operatory Thought in Piagetian theory is any procedure for mentally acting on objects. The hallmark of the preoperational stage is sparse and logically inadequate mental operations. During this stage the child learns to use and to represent objects by images and words, in other words they learn to use symbolic thinking. Thinking is still egocentric: The child has difficulty taking the viewpoint of others.

The child can classify objects by a single feature: e.g. groups together all the red blocks regardless of shape or all the square blocks regardless of colour. According to Piaget, the Pre-Operational stage of development follows the Sensorimotor stage and occurs between 2–7 years of age. In this stage, children develop their language skills.

They begin representing things with words and images. However, they still use intuitive rather than logical reasoning. At the beginning of this stage, they tend to be egocentric, that is, they are not aware that other people do not think, know and perceive the same as them. Children have highly imaginative minds at this time and actually assign emotions to inanimate objects. The theory of mind is also critical to this stage.

The Preoperational Stage can be further broken down into the Preconceptual Stage and the Intuitive.

The Preconceptual stage (2-4 years) is marked by egocentric thinking and animistic thought. A child who displays animistic thought tends to assign living attributes to inanimate objects, for example that a glass would feel pain if it were broken.

The Intuitive (4-7 years) stage is when children start employing mental activities to solve problems and obtain goals but they are unaware of how they came to their conclusions. For example a child is shown 7 dogs and 3 cats and asked if there are more dogs then cats. The child would respond positively. However when asked if there are more dogs then animals the child would once again respond positively. Such fundamental errors in logic show the transition between intuitiveness in solving problems and true logical reasoning acquired in later years. (Child Psychology, 1st Canadian Edition, Hetherington, Parke & Schmuckler).

Concrete Operational Stage

The Concrete operational stage is the third of four stages of cognitive development in Piaget's theory. This stage, which follows the Preoperational stage, occurs between the ages of 6 and 12 years and is characterized by the appropriate use of logic. Important processes during this stage are:

Seriation—the ability to sort objects in an order according to size, shape, or any other characteristic. For example, if given different-shaded objects they may make a colour gradient.

Classification—the ability to name and identify sets of objects according to appearance, size or other characteristic, including the idea that one set of objects can include another. A child is no longer subject to the illogical limitations of animism (the belief that all objects are alive and therefore have feelings).

Decentering—where the child takes into account multiple aspects of a problem to solve it. For example, the child will no longer perceive an exceptionally wide but short cup to contain less than a normally-wide, taller cup.

Reversibility—where the child understands that numbers or objects can be changed, then returned to their original state. For this reason, a child will be able to rapidly determine that if 4+4 equals 8, 8"4 will equal 4, the original quantity.

Conservation—understanding that quantity, length or number of items is unrelated to the arrangement or appearance of the object or items. For instance, when a child is presented with two equally-sized, full cups they will be able to discern that if water is transferred to a pitcher it will conserve the quantity and be equal to the other filled cup.

Elimination of Egocentrism—the ability to view things from another's perspective (even if they think incorrectly). For instance, show a child a comic in which Jane puts a doll under a box, leaves the room, and then Melissa moves the doll to a drawer, and Jane comes back. A child in the concrete operations stage will say that Jane will still think it's under the box even though the child knows it is in the drawer.

Formal Operational Stage

The formal operational period is the fourth and final of the periods of cognitive development in Piaget's theory. This stage, which follows the Concrete Operational stage, commences at around 11 years of age (puberty) and continues into adulthood. It is characterized by acquisition of the ability to think abstractly, reason logically and draw conclusions from the information available. During this stage the young adult is able to understand such things as love, "shades of gray", logical proofs, and values. Lucidly, biological factors may be traced to this stage as it occurs during puberty (the time at which another period of neural pruning occurs), marking the entry to adulthood in Physiology, cognition, moral judgment (Kohlberg), Psychosexual development (Freud), and social development (Erikson). Some two-thirds of people do not develop this form of reasoning fully enough that it becomes their normal mode for cognition, and so they remain, even as adults, concrete operational thinkers.

General Information Regarding the Stages

These four stages have been found to have the following characteristics:

- Although the timing may vary, the sequence of the stages does not.
- Universal (not culturally specific)
- Generalizable: the representational and logical operations available to the child should extend to all kinds of concepts and content knowledge
- Stages are logically organized wholes
- Hierarchical nature of stage sequences (each successive stage incorporates elements of previous stages, but is more differentiated and integrated)
- Stages represent qualitative differences in modes of thinking, not merely quantitative differences

Challenges to Piagetian Stage Theory

Piagetians accounts of development have been challenged on several grounds. First, as Piaget himself noted, development does not always progress in the smooth manner his theory seems to predict. 'Decalage', or unpredicted gaps in the developmental progression, suggest that the stage model is at best a useful approximation.

More broadly, Piaget's theory is 'domain general', predicting that cognitive maturation occurs concurrently across different domains of knowledge (such as mathematics, logic, understanding of physics, of language, etc.). However, more recent cognitive developmentalists have been much influenced by trends in cognitive science away from domain generality and towards domain specificity or modularity of mind, under which different cognitive faculties may be largely independent of one another and thus develop according to quite different timetables.

In this vein, many current cognitive developmentalists argue that rather than being domain general learners, children come equipped with domain specific theories, sometimes referred to as 'core knowledge', which allows them to break into learning within that domain. For example, even young infants appear to understand some basic principles of physics (e.g. that one object cannot pass through another) and human intention (e.g. that a hand repeatedly reaching for an object has that object, not just a particular path of motion, as its goal). These basic assumptions may be the building block out of which more elaborate knowledge is constructed.

Post Piagetian and Neo-Piagetian Stages

There are three major changes to the number of stages and their definitions. First and foremost, the half stages are now shown to be stages. Pascual Leone discovered this. Almost all Post Piagetians accept this. Second, postformal stages have been shown to exist. Kurt Fischer suggested two, Michael Commons presents evidence for four postformal stages: the systematic, metasystematic, paradigmatic and cross paradigmatic. Fischer has considered a stage suggested by Biggs and Biggs. It is a stage before the early preoperational. Commons and Richards call this stage the sentential because organisms can sequence representations of concepts.

Bruner's Thoery

Jerome S. Bruner (b. 1 October 1915) is an American psychologist, who has contributed to cognitive psychology and cognitive learning theory in educational psychology. Bruner's ideas are based on categorization. "To perceive is to categorize, to conceptualize is to categorize, to learn is to form categories, to make decisions is to categorize." Bruner maintains people interpret the world in terms of its similarities and differences. Like Bloom's Taxonomy, Bruner suggests a system of coding in which people form a hierarchical arrangement of related categories. Each successively higher level of categories becomes more specific, echoing Benjamin Bloom's understanding of knowledge acquisition as well as the related idea of instructional scaffolding. He has also suggested that there are two primary modes of thought: the narrative mode and the paradigmatic mode. In narrative thinking, the mind engages in sequential, action-oriented, detail-driven thought. In paradigmatic thinking, the mind transcends particularities to achieve systematic, categorical cognition. In the former case, thinking takes the form of stories and "gripping drama." In the latter, thinking is structured as propositions linked by logical operators.

The Narrative Construction of Reality

In 1991, Bruner published an article in *Critical Inquiry* entitled "The Narrative Construction of Reality." In this article, he argued that the mind structures its sense of reality through mediation through "cultural products, like language and other symbolic systems" (3). He specifically focuses on the idea of narrative as one of these cultural products. He defines narrative in terms of ten things:

1. Narrative diachronicity: The notion that narratives take place over some sense of time.
2. Particularity: The idea that narratives deal with particular events, although some events may be left vague and general.
3. Intentional state entailment: The concept that characters within a narrative have "beliefs, desires, theories, values, and so on" (7).

4. Hermeneutic composability: The theory that narratives are that which can be interpreted in terms of their role as a selected series of events that constitute a "story."
5. Canonicity and breach: The claim that stories are about something unusual happening that "breaches" the canonical (i.e. normal) state.
6. Referentiality: The principle that a story in some way references reality, although not in a direct way that offers verisimilitude.
7. Genericness: The flipside to particularity, this is the characteristic of narrative whereby the story can be classified as a genre.
8. Normativeness: The observation that narrative in some way supposes a claim about how one ought to act. This follows from canonicity and breach.
9. Context sensitivity and negotiability: Related to hermeneutic composability, this is the characteristic whereby narrative requires a negotiated role between author or text and reader, including the assigning of a context to the narrative, and ideas like suspension of disbelief.
10. Narrative accrual: Finally, the idea that stories are cumulative, that is, that new stories follow from older ones.

Bruner observes that these ten characteristics at once describe narrative and the reality constructed and posited by narrative, which in turn teaches us about the nature of reality as constructed by the human mind via narrative.

Jerome S Bruner's View about Cognitive Development of a Child

We have already discussed in details of the cognitive development of a child with special emphasis on Jean Piaget's views. So this is just a follow-up to that post with special reference to Jerome S. Burner.

Bruner, a renowned educational psychologist and Professor of Psychology at the New York University made a detailed study of cognitive development of the child and had suggested the following three stages.

- **Enactive Action:** It implies that most of the activities of the child are motor activities and are related to motor nerves.
- **Iconic Image:** At this stage the child is guided by his mental imagery. He is able to form his own mental images and expresses himself on that basis.
- **Symbolic Word**: The child at this stage expresses himself in the form of words. He comes to have a mental sense of time and distance. At this stage language learning also begin.

Conclusions

- The theory of Bruner resembles the theory of Piaget. The theory of Bruner is also more applicable during the period of infancy and childhood of the child.
- The teacher should utilize the internal imagery development of the child for his educational purposes. This mental imagery of the child would enable him in the conversation of his experiences and forge ahead with new experiences.

Concept Maps

A **concept map** is a diagram showing the relationships among concepts. They are graphical tools for organizing and representing knowledge. They include concepts, usually enclosed in circles or boxes of some type, and relationships between concepts indicated by a connecting line linking two concepts. Concepts can be connected with labelled arrows, in a downward-branching hierarchical structure. The relationship between concepts can be articulated in linking phrases, e.g., "gives rise to", "results in", "is required by," or "contributes to". The technique for visualizing these relationships among different concepts is called *Concept mapping.*

Overview

A concept map is a way of representing relations between ideas, images or words, in the same way that a sentence diagram represents the grammar of a sentence, a road map represents the locations of highways and towns, and a circuit diagram represents the workings of an electrical appliance. In a concept map, each word or phrase is connected to another and linked back to the original idea, word or phrase. Concept maps are a way to develop logical thinking and study skills, by revealing connections and helping students see how individual ideas form a larger whole. Concept maps were developed to enhance meaningful learning in the sciences. A well made concept map grows within a *context frame* defined by an explicit "focus question," while a mind map often has only branches radiating out from a central picture. There is research evidence that knowledge is stored in the brain in the form of productions that act on declarative memory content which is also referred to as chunks or propositions. Because concept maps are constructed to reflect the organization of the declarative memory system, they facilitate sense-making and meaningful learning on the part of individuals who make concept maps and those who use them.

Concept mapping can be contrasted with the similar idea of mind mapping, which is often restricted to radial hierarchies and tree structures. Among the various schema and techniques for visualizing ideas, processes, organizations, concept mapping, as developed by Novak is unique in philosophical basis, which "makes concepts, and propositions composed of concepts, the central elements in the structure of knowledge and construction of meaning." Another contrast between Concept mapping and Mind mapping is the speed and spontaneity when a Mind map is created. A Mind map reflects what you think about a single topic, which can focus group brainstorming. A Concept map can be a map, a system view, of a real (abstract) system or set of concepts. Concept maps are more free form, as multiple hubs and clusters can be created, unlike mindmaps which fix on a single conceptual centre.

Sociable Thinking: Cognitive Development in Early Childhood Education

In a review of cognitive development written in 1993, I wrote that I wanted to promote breadth and flexibility of perspective: there are different theories and informal views of thinking, I said, each with advantages and problems for early childhood educators (Seifert, 1993). Theoretical changes in the intervening years, however, have made me regard this liberal, tolerant view as naive. New models of cognitive development and their embodiments in early childhood education have moved markedly toward socially based theories of learning (SBTLs), theories variously called social constructivism, socio-historical perspectives, or (less accurately) simply constructivism. In some circles, SBTLs now verge on taken-as-given, universal "truths"-something of an oxymoron given their constructivist premises!

So my challenge as a reviewer has shifted. I still want to avoid "theoretical sectarianism" about cognitive development, but I especially want to avoid evangelizing too hard for the dominant constructivist "churches"-to avoid accepting SBTLs too easily, without critical appraisal. Accomplishing this new task can be challenging, given the support for SBTLs circulating in the current post-modernist Zeitgeist. Nonetheless, my hope in this chapter is to encourage an appraisal of SBTLs both directly and indirectly by describing aspects of SBTLs and alternatives theories, and the commenting on what each offers early childhood education and on how much each is partaking of the "new" constructivisms. The appraisals will not aim for full coverage, but emphasize the practical needs of early childhood educators, who I will define as any professionals who work with and support children day-to-day, regardless of institutional affiliation.

I will describe four major theories or models related to cognitive development in early childhood. The first will be learning theory, but learning theory primarily in its recent, relatively cognitive versions. The second will be information processing theory, with special emphasis on the newer ideas about pattern detection and parallel, rather than serial, processing. The third will be structural theory, with emphasis on what might be termed the "organizing inner mind." The fourth will be SBTLs proper, in both individualistic and social forms. This sequence will work, but not perfectly, because versions of SBTL have influenced all schools of developmental thought and early childhood education practice. The problem, it will turn out, is that distinctions among theories and concepts are not fully stable or clear. Blurring conceptual and pedagogical boundaries has mostly been healthy, but the reasons for blurrings need to be understood carefully, in order to make best use of the revisions in daily work with children.

To help fix the conceptual distinctions and shifts, I begin by discussing my understanding of what psychologists and educators tend to mean by the general term cognitive development, and its relevance (or lack thereof) for early childhood education. As we will see, the notion ofcognitive development is problematic for early childhood educators because it implies psychological distinctions not held by them in practice, or even in published reflections on their work. But the mismatch between "classic" cognitive development and the needs of professionals has apparently been noticed by developmental psychologists, some of whom have revised their research projects to bring them more in line with (and also help to create) newer meanings ofcognitive development. For better or for worse, the new meanings are all more socially based or "social constructivist" than before; hence my cautions in the opening paragraph of this chapter.

Learning Theory as Cognitive Development

Traditionally, learning theory has focused on forms of human change that were by definition somewhat peripheral to human development. Learning theory was about relatively rapid associations between stimuli or between responses and reinforcements. When stimuli, responses and consequences were all simple enough and when conditions were properly controlled, the fast-paced (by developmental standards) stimuli and responses displayed lawful properties and allowed for testable predictions about (short-term) behaviour change. The resulting changes were called "learning." Connections between stimuli were named associative learning or "classical" conditioning, and those between a response and its consequence were named operant conditioning. Those between a response and consequence that were merely observed by an individual were called Modelling, observational learning or "vicarious conditioning."

Assessed in terms of developmental theory and of SBTL, the problem with behaviourally oriented learning theory had three blind spots: it did not say enough about long-term change, about the experience of learning, or about how learning and behaviour became organized in the minds and lives of learners. Observational learning theory was an early effort to remedy the last two of the three problems (Bandura, 1977), and represented an initial turn toward what SBTL theorists eventually called meaning-making. In observational learning, a person somehow "sees" relationships between a relatively complex behaviour and its consequences. A student does not merely see a classmate elevate an arm and vocalize, for example, but sees the classmate "answer a teacher's question." If the teacher then tightens facial muscles, the student sees not merely muscular action, but sees the teacher "smile in response to the student." In observational learning theory, observed concrete behaviours become expressions of meanings perceived as happening in others (Bandura, 1995). This approach is still far from the thorny issues of interpretation discussed by social constructivists, but it is nonetheless a nod toward students' lived experience and personally constructed meanings.

Recent versions of learning theory have moved even more toward meaning-making than did Bandura and his colleagues. In one relatively radical formulation of learning theory, for example, conditioning has been interpreted as not about behaviour change per se, but about making meaning (DeGrandpre, 2000). In this view, linkages among overt stimulus cues, responses and consequences are merely cases of this broader process. Operant conditioning is not merely about reinforcing or strengthening specific responses as a result of specific consequences, but about creating perceived relationships among responses, the stimuli prior to responses, and the consequences that follow. "Reinforcement" of a behaviour is therefore not simply the consequences of a behaviour, as in earlier versions of learning theory, but the relationship among all elements of a learning trial-stimuli, responses, and consequences. If a teacher smiles pleasantly at a young child's interesting comment during a circle-time discussion, for example, what is reinforced is not just the child's tendency to make verbal comments in the future. What is reinforced is actually the child's tendency to associate or connect the teacher's smile, the child's own verbal contributions, and the setting or conditions when doing so is appropriate. To say that "the teacher reinforces the child with her smile," in fact is misleading because it implies more control on the part of the teacher than the teacher really has. She does contribute to the reinforcement-relationship by smiling, but so do the classroom circumstances and the child's own behaviour. All must happen together, and together they constitute reinforcement-and the creation of meaning.

Learning theory has also become more constructivist by developing more complex models of how children learn, and therefore more able to explain concepts and skills that truly matter in the lives of children and caregivers. An example is the "overlapping waves theory" proposed recently by Robert Siegler (1996). This theory makes three assumptions: 1) that children normally use a variety of strategies for solving problems, 2) that strategies can co-exist for long periods even when some are suboptimal or incompatible, and 3) that experience changes the relative salience of particular strategies, rather than eliminating any outright. Changes in salience alter the likelihood of particular strategies actually appearing as behaviour. When graphed across time, relative salience rises and falls like a series of overlapping waves; hence the name of the model. Learning theory-or at least Siegler's overlapping waves version of learning theory-is about studying these changes in salience and their eventual expression as altered behaviour.

The result, compared to older models of learning, are predictions about learning that are more realistic. In actual classroom practice, a child is indeed likely to try a variety of strategies in ways that are often somewhat trial-and-error. A child may work two-digit subtraction problems, for example, by using "borrowing" algorithms officially recommended by the teacher, but also persist in counting on fingers some of the time, and at other times also try personalized (often bug-ridden) one-digit procedures that work only with particular subsets of problems. Even when a child gains skill with a new strategy-in this case the "borrowing" algorithm-he or she still often regresses to earlier methods now and then, just as adults do. The child is sometimes also likely to spend time perfecting existing, suboptimal approaches rather than trying new ones-learning to count on fingers faster or more surreptitiously, for example-since doing so usually has short-term payoff. New, more optimal strategies appear both suddenly and intermittently when and if they finally do. The relative importance of a child's alternative subtraction strategies will gradually change with practice, but suboptimal ones will not totally disappear for quite a while, if ever. The results are patterns of behaviour that resemble Siegler's "overlapping waves" model of learning (Siegler, 2000).

The educational value of a more meaning-oriented version of learning theory can be seen in the recent professional writing of early educators. Discussions of behaviour problems in young children, for example, still draw heavily on concepts of applied behaviour analysis (Kaiser and Rasminsky, 1999; Scarlett, 1998). Teachers are often still urged to frame behaviour problems in terms of operant conditioning (or as antecedents, behaviour, and consequences, which amount to the same idea), in order to influence a child's unwanted behaviour.

But though this literature is quite behaviourist, it often is also concerned with the meaning of antecedents, behaviour, and consequences for the child: with the relationships she perceives among these elements, and with how a teacher might influence the perceptions in desirable directions. One result is that teachers are urged to alter not just consequences, but also the connections (or lack thereof) among antecedents, behaviour, and consequences. A temper tantrum may be highly disruptive, for example, but the solution may not be simply to avoid paying attention to it (withholding reinforcement in the narrow sense). It may also be necessary to avoid connecting antecedents to the tantrum behaviours-avoid the triggers for tantrums in the first place. Not only is the broader strategy more likely to alter behaviour, it is also more likely to help a child "see" his tantrum in new, more acceptable ways-to alter, that is, its personal meaning.

Much of the literature on behaviour management also implies a learning theory of "overlapping waves." In discussing how to deal with a tantrum, for example, teachers are reminded that relapses are likely to occur, and that teachers should persevere with altering relationships among antecedents, responses, and consequences in spite of them. Expecting relapses implies that a child is guided by competing responses that are gradually shifting in relative importance or salience. Helping a child respond to frustration in consistently desirable ways is really a matter of developing a high ratio of desirable responses to undesirable ones, and thereby also making the desirable responses highly "meaningful" to the child in the sense of strengthening their connections to antecedents and consequences.

In addition to becoming more compatible with early childhood practice, such revisions to learning theory have had significant influences both on learning theory itself and on traditional meanings of human development, including cognitive development. The ideas about meaningful reinforcement described earlier bring learning theory closer to SBTLs in that it becomes more concerned than before about how learning is experienced by the child and how the child can take responsibility for "constructing" new, learned behaviours. The shifting, overlapping strategies described by Siegler, on the other hand, blur the conventional distinction between short- and long-term change which has been central to the idea of cognitive development. At the heart of the model is a process that is continuous, yet never complete, and in this sense it is neither short-nor long-term, but always both and always lifelong.

Mingling the short-and long-term is consistent with the professional needs of teachers and others with direct responsibilities for children. As professionals, we are fundamentally concerned with connecting the past and the future to a child's present: with helping children to relate previous experience and future intentions to current skills and plans. Classroom practice can be interpreted, in fact, as an active effort to combine the short-term (the current activity) with the long-term (the child's prior skills and knowledge with the child's goals), even though doing so confuses the conventional distinction between immediate learning and long-term growth implied by the term cognitive development. In addition, of course, good teaching of the young integrates children's actions in other ways. Teachers often attend to a child's unstated intuitions and fully conscious reasoning simultaneously; or they deal with a child's individual academic achievements and social relationships at the same time. In order to understand these concerns in parallel, integrated ways, even the revised versions of learning theory are not fully helpful, and early childhood educators must again turn elsewhere, such as to information processing theory or to SBTL itself. The next section considers the first of these alternatives, information processing theory, and its relation to cognitive development and to early childhood education. Following this discussion, we can look directly at what SBTLs have to offer.

Imagery—Language and Thinking

Imagery, Language and Visuo-Spatial Thinking discusses the remarkable human ability to use mental imagery in everyday life: from helping plan actions and routes to aiding creative thinking; from making sense of and remembering our immediate environment to generating pictures in our minds from verbal descriptions of scenes or people. The book also considers the important theme of how individuals differ in their ability to use imagery. With contributions from leading researchers in the field, this book will be of interest to advanced undergraduates, postgraduates and researchers in cognitive psychology, cognitive science and cognitive neuropsychology.

Reasoning and Problem Solving—Implications to the Teacher

Reasoning

Humans have the ability to engage in reasoning about their own reasoning. Different forms of such reflection on reasoning occur in different fields. In philosophy, the study of reasoning typically focuses on what makes reasoning efficient or inefficient, appropriate or inappropriate, good or bad. Philosophers do this by either examining the form or structure of the reasoning within arguments, or by considering the broader methods used to reach particular goals of reasoning. Psychologists and cognitive scientists, in contrast, tend to study how people reason, which cognitive and neural processes are engaged, how cultural factors affect the inferences people draw. The properties of logics which may be used to reason are studied in mathematical logic. The field of automated reasoning studies how reasoning may be modelled computationally. Lawyers also study reasoning.

Problem Solving

Problem solving forms part of thinking. Considered the most complex of all intellectual functions, problem solving has been defined as higher-order cognitive process that requires the modulation and control of more routine or fundamental skills. It occurs if an organism or an artificial intelligence system does not know how to proceed from a given state to a desired goal state. It is part of the larger problem process that includes problem finding and problem shaping.

Problem solving is of crucial importance in engineering when products or processes fail, so corrective action can be taken to prevent further failures. Perhaps of more value, problem solving can be applied to a product or process prior to an actual fail event i.e. a potential problem can be predicted, analyzed and mitigation applied so the problem never actually occurs. Techniques like Failure Mode Effects Analysis can be used to proactively reduce the likelihood of problems occurring. Forensic engineering is an important technique of failure analysis which involves tracing product defects and flaws. Corrective action can then be taken to prevent further failures.

Unit-IV

Social, Emotional and Moral Development

Social Development

Social development is a process which results in the transformation of social structures in a manner which improves the capacity of the society to fulfil its aspirations. Society develops by consciousness and social consciousness develops by organization. The process that is subconscious in the society emerges as conscious knowledge in pioneering individuals. Development is a process, not a programme. Its power issues more from its subtle aspects than from material objects.

Not all social change constitutes development. It consists of four well-marked stages — survival, growth, development and evolution, each of which contains the other three within it. The quantitative expansion of existing activities generates growth or horizontal expansion. Development implies a qualitative change in the way the society carries out its activities, such as through more progressive attitudes and behaviour by the population, the adoption of more effective social organizations or more advanced technology which may have been developed elsewhere. The term evolution refers to the original formulation and adoption of qualitative and structural advances in the form of new social attitudes, values, behaviours, or organizations.

While the term is usually applied to changes that are beneficial to society, it may result in negative side-effects or consequences that undermine or eliminate existing ways of life that are considered positive.

Factors of Social Developments

Discrimination: Sometimes there are social or cultural factors that hold back poor countries. Discrimination is one of these. If there are certain people groups that are discriminated against, the country's overall productivity can suffer. This may be a tribe, a caste, a racial category or minority language group. I have already mentioned Cameroon, which has both French speaking and English speaking regions. All the infrastructure happens in the French speaking part. French speakers in Canada complain of the opposite. Welsh speakers in Britain, or Catalans in Spain, have historically faced similar problems. Racial discrimination may be an issue, excluding certain groups from economic activity, either deliberately or not. Racial minorities regularly have poorer exam results and economic prospects than the majority. More serious forms of exclusion would be apartheid South Africa, or the Asian communities driven out of Uganda under Idi Amin, which was disastrous for Uganda's economy.

Another division may be the role of women. Jeffrey Sachs talks about this in The End of Poverty: 'Cultural or religious norms may block the role of women... leaving half the population without economic or political rights and without education, thereby undermining half of the population in its contribution to overall development.' If you don't believe that women should work, you have effectively halved the earning potential of your country.

Population: Closely linked to this is the population issue. If women see staying at home and bringing up children as their chief role, they will have more children than those who work. There is nothing wrong with having lots of children, as long as you can provide for them. Jeffrey Sachs again: 'With fewer children, a poor household can invest more in the health and education of each child, thereby equipping the next generation with the health, nutrition, and education that can lift living standards in future years.'

As Paul has talked about here before, world population has exploded. What is interesting is that the countries where this has happened are often those where women do not play a role in business or society. When women are educated and given a choice, some will stay at home and look after children, and others will pursue careers or start small businesses.

This is an important factor, as some countries have seen their population double or triple without their economies keeping pace. That leaves more mouths to feed, and just not enough to go around.

Culture

I've already mentioned the role of women, but culture can have hidden effects in business, trade and development. China may be a major power now, but it was the world's most developed country in the middle ages, and stagnated, or even went backwards, for centuries. Part of this was cultural, a pride and sense of self-sufficiency that led to a closing of China's borders. 'China seems to have long been stationary', Adam Smith wrote in 1776, in his Wealth of Nations. 'A country which neglects or despises foreign commerce... cannot transact the same quantity of business which it might do with different laws and institutions.' That's changed, but nationalism, suspicion, or radical philosophy still has some countries closed down to outside involvement – communism in North Korea, or extremist Islam in Taliban Afghanistan, locking countries out of development.

This the far end of the spectrum, but culture works in subtler ways too. Some cultures believe in a greater good, in unity, in the rule of law. They are optimistic, hopeful, ambitious and ready to pull together. Others can be paranoid, fragmented, uncertain of their place in the modern world, angry, resistant to change.

Rich countries can be overconfident and brash. Poor countries can see themselves as victims and become despondent. In his The Wealth and Poverty of Nations, economic historian David Landes says 'If we learn anything from the history of economic development it is that culture makes all the difference.'

Social Maturity: Erikson's Stages of Social Development

What we've just gone over is a sort of abstracted version of Kegan's social maturity theory without any real detail shown. Of course, it will help to have that detail along with some concrete examples of what he is talking about to make this all comprehensible, so that is what I will now try to supply.

Kegan is suggesting that as babies grow into adults, they develop progressively more objective and accurate appreciations of the social world they inhabit. They do this by progressing through five or more states or periods of development which he labelled as follows:

- Incorporative
- Impulsive
- Imperial
- Interpersonal
- Institutional.

In their beginnings, babies are all subjective and have really no appreciation of anything objective at all, and therefore no real self-awareness. This is to say, at first, babies have little idea how to interpret anything, and the only perspective they have with which to interpret things is their own scarcely developed perspective. They can recognize parent's faces and the like, but this sort of recognition should not be confused with babies being able to appreciate that parents are separate creatures with their own needs. This key recognition doesn't occur for years.

Kegan describes this earliest period as **Incorporative**. The sense of self is not developed at this point in time. There is no self to speak of because there is no distinction occurring yet between self and other. To the baby, there is not any reason to ask the question, "who am I" because the baby's mind is nothing more and nothing less than the experience of its senses as it moves about. In an important sense, the baby is embedded in its sensory experience and has no other awareness.

Babies practice using their senses and reflexes a lot and thus develop mental representations of those reflexes. At some point it occurs to the baby that it *has* reflexes that it can use and senses that it can experience. Reflex and sensation are thus the first mental objects; the first things that are understood to be distinct components of the self. The sense of self emerges from the knowledge that there are things in the world that aren't self (like reflexes and senses); things that I am not. To quote Kegan,

> *"Rather than literally being my reflexes, I now have them, and "I" am something other. "I" am that which coordinates or mediates the reflexes..."*

Kegan correspondingly refers to this second period of social appreciation development as **Impulsive**, to suggest that the child is now embedded in impulses – which are those things that coordinate reflexes. The sense of self at this stage of life would be comfortable saying something like, "hungry", or "sleepy", being fully identified with these hungers. Though babies are now aware that they can take action to fulfil a need, they still are not clear that other people exist yet as independent creatures. From the perspective of the Impulsive mind, a parent is merely another reflex that can be brought to bear to satisfy impulses.

The objectification of what was previously subjective experience continues as development continues. Kegan's next developmental leap is known as the **Imperial** self. The child as "little dictator" is born. In the prior impulsive self, the self literally is nothing more and nothing less than a set of needs. *There isn't anyone "there" having those needs yet. The needs alone are all that exists.* As awareness continues to rise, the child now starts to become aware that "it" is the very thing that has the needs. Because the child is now aware that it *has* needs (rather than *is* needs), it also starts to become aware that it can consciously manipulate things to get its needs satisfied. The impulsive child was also manipulative, perhaps, but in a more unaware animal manner. The imperial child is not yet aware that other people have needs too. It only knows at this stage that it has needs, and it doesn't hesitate to express them.

The **Interpersonal** period that follows next starts with the first moment when the child comes to understand that there are actually other people out there in the world whose needs need to be taken into account along side their own. The appreciation of the otherness of other people comes about, as always by a process of expanding perspectives. The child's perspective in this case expands from its own only to later include both its own and those of other important people around it. It is the child's increasingly sophisticated understanding of the idea that people have needs itself which cause the leap to occur. To quote Kegan again,

> *"I" no longer am my needs (no longer the imperial I); rather I have them. In having them I can now coordinate, or integrate, one need system with another, and in so doing, I bring into being that need-mediating reality which we refer to when we speak of mutuality."*

In English then, the interpersonal child becomes aware that "not only do I have needs, *other people do too!*" This moment in time is where conscience is born and the potential for guilt and shame arises, as well as the potential for empathy. Prior to this moment, these important aspects of adult mental life don't exist except as potentials.

The interpersonal child is aware that other people have needs which it needs to be taken into account if it is to best satisfy its own needs. There is no guiding principle that helps the interpersonal child to determine which set of needs is most important – its own, or those of the other people. Some children will conclude that their own needs are most important to satisfy, while others will conclude that other's needs should be prioritized, and some children will move back and forth between the two positions like a crazy monkey.

As the child's sense of self continues to develop, at some point it becomes aware that a guiding principle can be established which helps determine which set of needs should take precedence under particular circumstances. This is the first moment that the child can be said to have values, or commitments to ideas and beliefs and principles which are larger and more permanent than its own passing whims and fears. Kegan refers to this new realization of and commitment to values as the **Institutional** period, noting that in this period, the child's idea of self becomes something which can be, for the first time, described in terms of institutionalized values, such as being honest. "I'm an honest person. I try to be fair. I strive to be brave." are the sorts of things an institutional mind might say. Values, such as the Golden Rule (e.g., "Do unto others as you would have them do unto you"), start to guide the child's appreciation of how to be a member of the family and of society. The moral, ethical and legal foundations of society follow from this basic achievement of an Institutional self. Further, children (or adults) who achieve this level of social maturity understand the need for laws and for ethical codes that work to govern everyone's behaviour. Less socially mature individuals won't grasp why these things are important and cannot and should not simply be disregarded when they are inconvenient.

For many people, social maturity seems to stop here at the Institutional stage. Kegan himself writes that this stage is the stage of conventional adult maturity; one that many (but not all) adults reach, and beyond which most do not progress. However, the potential for continued development continues onwards and upwards.

The next evolution of self understanding occurs when the child (by now probably an adult) starts to realize that there is more than one way of being "fair" or "honest" or "brave" in the world. Whereas before, in the interpersonal mindset, there is only one possible right way to interpret a social event (e.g., in accordance with one's own value system), a newly developed **Inter-industrial** mindset starts to recognize a diversity of ways that someone might act and still be acting in accordance with a coherent value system (though not necessarily one's own value system).

For example, let's consider how someone with an Institutional mindset and someone with an InterIndividual mindset might judge someone who has become a "draft dodger" so as to avoid military duty. There are precisely two ways that an Institutionally minded person might look at such an action. If he or she is of the mainstream institutional mindset, draft dodging is a non-religious sort of heresy and a crime which should be punishable. If, on the other hand, he or she is of a counter-cultural institutional mindset, then judgements are reversed and draft dodging is seen as a brave action which demonstrates individual courage in the face of massive peer pressure to conform. An institutionally minded person can hold *one or the other* of these perspectives but not both, because he or she is literally embedded in one or the other of those perspectives and cannot appreciate the other except as something alien and evil.

A person who has achieved InterIndividual social maturity is able to hold both mainstream and counter-cultural value systems in mind at the same time, and to see the problem of draft dodging from both perspectives. This sort of dual-vision will appear to be the worst kind of wishy-washiness and flip-floppery to someone stuck in a conventional Institutional mindset and maturity level. However, if you are following the progression of social maturity states, and how one states' embedded subjective view becomes something which is seem objectively alongside other points of view as social maturity progresses, you will see that such dual-vision is indeed the logical next step; what a more socially mature sort of human being might look like.

Kegan thinks of the achievement of InterIndividual social maturity, what might be considered "post-maturity", as a dubious thing. In a wonderful interview published by "What is Enlightenment Magazine " and available online here, Kegan comments on the danger that this state poses:

> *"... you have to think about what it means to actually be more complex than what your culture is currently demanding. You have to have a name for that, too. It's almost something beyond maturity, and it's usually a very risky state to be in. I mean, we loved Jesus, Socrates, and Gandhi—after we murdered them. While they were alive, they were a tremendous pain in the ass. Jesus, Abraham Lincoln, Martin Luther King, Jr.—these people died relatively young. You don't often live a long life being too far out ahead of your culture."*

I'm not going to comment on whether or not Kegan's social maturity theory is accurate. Whether or not it is accurate, it is still a very useful and interesting way of thinking about how social maturity develops. If we can agree to accept this theory as basically correct, for a moment, a whole lot of mental problems and disorders that are otherwise difficult to talk about suddenly start to make some sense; start to "click into place". This is already a rather long essay and I don't want to belabour it, but I need to give at least one example, and to my mind there is no better example for my purpose than Narcissistic Personality Disorder.

Narcissists are (typically) arrogant, self-important and even grandiose people who consider themselves special and "above the law", lacking in empathy and compassion, willing to exploit innocents, and who are consumed by visions of dramatic personal success and power to which they quite passionately believe they are entitled for no apparent reason. Narcissists use other people if it suits their purpose to use them, and discard or attack them if they are in the way.

Everyone knows a few people who fit the narcissist mold to one degree or another. It is generally not at all clear what the heck is wrong with narcissists that causes them to act in this obnoxious fashion, so most people tend to think of them in more simple terms, as "jerks" or "a holes".

Now, think for a moment what an adult might look like who never left the Imperial self stage of social maturity development. Keep in mind that there are many different types of maturity and that we are only suggesting an adult whose growth has been stunted in this particular social-emotional manner. Other aspects of maturity (e.g., cognitive and intellectual maturity, knowledge, and of course age) are unaffected. That particular hypothetical adult is pretty much going to look like a narcissist, huh? A "little dictator" writ into adult form.

For example, the adult narcissist lacks empathy for the same reason that the normal imperial child lacks empathy; as an Imperially minded individual, he cannot conceive of any perspective that has any meaning other than his own. He or she is literally embedded in an inadequate and inaccurate representation of social reality; one in which only his own needs and impulses are important and no one else is important.

The existence of other human beings with separate needs may be partially understood by such a fellow, but there is no recognition that those other people's needs have equivalent weight and reality to the Imperial-minded narcissists' own.

A similar argument can be made to explain how to account for sociopaths; antisocial personality disorders (who similarly lacks in empathy, guilt and remorse for criminal actions which harm other people), and also for the childish, immature and often reckless behaviour that is frequently displayed by otherwise normal people who have been abusing drugs and/or alcohol since they were small and have only recently become sober. Such people's behaviour can be made more comprehensible if you think of them as developmentally delayed in this dimension of social-emotional maturity.

Just because we can use Kegan's theory to explain why people act like jerks, doesn't for a second excuse jerky behaviour. Or criminal behaviour, for that matter. Adult narcissists and antisocials may be akin to little children in terms of their social maturity development, but they are not typically retarded in other aspects of maturity. They often have the full compliment of adult intellectual capabilities and may even have very good social skills. They often know right from wrong in some abstract manner even if they can't conceive it like a more socially mature person might. They are accountable for their actions even if they possess real handicaps that lead them to act in unacceptable ways.

Ask any therapist and he or she will tell you-it is quite difficult to do effective therapy with people who have social immaturity problems. If Kegan is right in his thinking, the reason for this would not be that these people are fundamentally resistant to the therapy process (which is how many therapists see the problem), but rather in large part because they cannot *comprehend* the therapy process, which is after all, very much a social process that requires a certain level of social maturity on the part of patients before they can benefit. It isn't enough to simply teach a set of skills to such people, because all such people will be capable of doing is aping those skills. They won't be able to fully appreciate the meaning of those skills and thus generalize from them to a more abstract (and mature) way of being with other people. Teaching social skills might actually work for some such people. Some people might actually learn the skills and that will be enough to trigger their growth. However, there ought to be a better, more direct way to make this sort of social maturity growth occur.

Actually, the question of how to help adult people become more socially mature when they aren't is a huge unanswered question that this theory leaves us with. Is there a way to help the Narcissists and the Antisocials and the Pedophiles out there? What about the rest of the people out there who are not quite at the level of social maturity that society demands of them? Kegan explores these questions in his follow-on book, In Over Our Heads" which is also very good and worth reading. If there is interest in this essay (we'll see), I'll find a way to go over his conclusions from that book in a future essay.

Hopefully, those of you who have stuck this out will have comprehended what I've been trying to say and it will have been a worthwhile expenditure of your time. If not, all I can say in my defense is that I tried my best (grin!). My aim is to educate, and this stuff is worth knowing about, even if it isn't something Oprah or Dr. Phil would do a show about. As per usual, I'm happy to answer questions and post non-trollish comments. Be well.

Emotional Development—Meaning—Positive and Negative Emotions

Research and theory on the role of emotion and regulation in morality have received considerable attention in the last decade. Much relevant work has concerned the role of moral emotions in moral behaviour. Research on differences between embarrassment, guilt, and shame and their relations to moral behaviour is reviewed, as is research on the association of these emotions with negative emotionality and regulation.

Recent issues concerning the role of such empathy-related responses as sympathy and personal distress to prosocial and antisocial behaviour are discussed, as is the relation of empathy-related responding to situational and dispositional emotionality and regulation. The development and socialization of guilt, shame, and empathy also are discussed briefly. In addition, the role of nonmoral emotions (e.g. anger and sadness), including moods and dispositional differences in negative emotionality and its regulation, in morally relevant behaviour, is reviewed.

Theories of Emotion

Several perspectives help explain the role of emotion in development. Some theorists emphasize that emotions occur during events involving self and environment, but that events must be cognitively appraised before an emotion is experienced; this appraisal occurs with reference to one's goals (Frijda, Kuipers, and ter Schure 1989; Lazarus 1991).

The *social constructivist* approach (e.g., Saarni 1999) also highlights appraisal, but focuses on emotions as social products based on cultural beliefs. In contrast, *Differential Emotions Theory* asserts that different emotions are already present at birth (Izard 1991). Keith Oatley and Jennifer Jenkins (1996) assimilate these divergent views, holding that emotions derive from a universal biological core, but also contain an appraisal/semantic component that is largely a product of social construction.

Emotional Competence

Both Susanne Denham (1998) and Carolyn Saarni (1990, 1999) have written about children's emotional competence; they agree that, although there are no overarching stages for emotional development, children become increasingly sophisticated in their expression and experience, understanding, and regulation of emotions. These early foundations of emotional competence contribute to mental health throughout the lifespan.

Socialization of emotional competence: Because emotions are inherently social, skills of emotional competence are vividly played out during interaction and within relationships with others. As noted by Joseph Campos and Karen Barrett (1984), emotions provide useful information for self and others. This entry focuses on the emotional transactions between parent and child and on parents' contributions to emotional competence.

Amy Halberstadt (1991) has highlighted three possible mechanisms of parents' socialization of emotional competence: Modelling, reactions to children's emotions, and teaching about emotions. The theories of psychologists like Sylvan Tomkins (1963, 1991), as well as empirical findings from late twentieth-century research (e.g., Denham, Cook and Zoller 1992; Denham and Kochanoff, in press; Denham et al. 1997; Denham, Zoller, and Couchoud 1994; Dunn, Brown, and Beardsall 1991; Eisenberg, Cumberland, and Spinrad 1998; Eisenberg and Fabes 1994; Eisenberg, Fabes, and Murphy 1996; Eisenberg et al. 1999), predict that parents' positive emotional expression and experience, accepting and helpful reactions to children's emotions, and emphasis on teaching about emotions in the family, contribute to young children's more sophisticated emotional competence.

Over and above these mechanisms for the socialization of emotion, cultural issues are paramount (e.g., Kitayama and Markus 1994; Lutz 1994; Markus and Kitayama 1994; Matsumoto 1994; Matsumoto et al. 1988; Saarni 1998; Shiraev and Levy 2001). Parents socialize their children based on specific cultural values and norms, but cross-cultural similarities and differences remain to be delineated. In both Japan and the United States, people often agree on the antecedents and evaluative components of emotional experience, and even on some primitive aspects of appraisal (e.g., "I was scared of the loud noise; that didn't feel good; it seemed certain that something bad was about to happen; I had to decide how to cope"). Nevertheless, they differ markedly on some of the more advanced aspects of appraisal, including control of and responsibility for emotion. In the United States, people might state, "I have to show this emotion," or even "I am not responsible for this emotion," whereas the Japanese might say "I should not show this emotion" and "I am responsible for this emotion" (Mauro, Sato, and Tucker 1992; Nakamura, Buck, and Kenny 1990). Given these differences, the goals of emotion socialization surely differ across the two cultures.

Regarding Modelling, children observe parents' ever-present emotions, and incorporate this learning into their expressive behaviour. Parents' expressiveness also teaches children which emotions are acceptable in which contexts. Their emotional displays tell children about the emotional significance of differing events, behaviours that may accompany differing emotions, and others' likely reactions. A mostly positive emotional family climate makes learning about emotions accessible to children (e.g., Garner, Jones, and Miner 1994). Thus, parents' expressiveness is associated with children's understanding of emotions as well as their expressiveness (Denham and Grout 1992, 1993; Denham, Zoller, and Couchoud 1994).

However, several factors suggest possible negative contributions of parents' expressiveness to children's emotional competence. Parents' frequent and intense negative emotions may disturb children, making emotional learning more difficult. Further, parents whose expressiveness is generally limited impart little information about emotions to their children (Denham, Zoller, and Couchoud 1994).

Parents may cultivate some emotional expressions, but not others. Western cultures urge children to separate self from others and express themselves, but many non-Western cultures view people as fundamentally connected, with the goal of socialization attunement or alignment of one's actions and reactions with that of others'. Thus, in Japan, the public display of emotions is mostly discouraged because it is seen as disruptive, leading us to expect Japanese parents to model mostly low intensity emotions (Ujiie 1997).

Moreover, there is a qualitative difference in the emotions modelled. Valued emotions accompanying interdependence—friendliness, affiliation, calmness, smoothness, and connectedness—would be most available for observation by Japanese children. In contrast, anger, regarded as extremely negative in Japan because it disturbs interdependence, would be modelled less (Ujiie 1997). Research on these culturally unique aspects of socialization of emotions, however, is still largely lacking.

Parents' contingent reactions to children's emotional displays are also linked to children's emotionally competent expression, experience, understanding, and regulation of emotions (Denham, Zoller, Couchoud 1994; Denham et al. 1997; Eisenberg and Fabes 1994; Eisenberg, Fabes, and Murphy 1996; Eisenberg et al. 1999). Contingent reactions include Behavioural and emotional encouragement or discouragement of specific emotions. Parents who dismiss emotions may actively punish children for showing emotions, or they may want to be helpful, but ignore their child's emotions in an effort to "make it better." Children who experience negative reactions are distressed by their parents' reactions as well as the events that originally elicited emotion.

Positive reactions, such as tolerance or comforting, convey a very different message—that emotions are manageable, even useful. Good emotion coaches, at least in the United States, accept children's experiences of emotion and their expression of emotions that do not harm others; they empathize with and validate emotions. In fact, emotional moments may be opportunities for parent-child intimacy (Gottman, Katz, and Hooven 1997).

Japanese parents' reactions to children's emotions differ from U.S. parents', although not at every age or in every situation. In general, U.S. parents *Children observe parents' emotions and incorporate this learning into their expressive behaviour. Parents' emotional displays tell children about the significance of events, behaviours that may accompany emotions, and others' likely reactions.* OWEN FRANKEN/CORBIS see expression of emotions as legitimate and part of healthy self-assertion. Japanese mothers also respond positively to their infants and young children's emotions (Kanaya, Nakamura, and Miyake 1989), but gradually emphasize, more than U.S. parents, parenting goals of *inhibitory self-regulation* and *acquisition of good manners.* Thus, for children older than about three years, Japanese mothers react most positively to children's suppression of emotion and demonstration of empathy. Compared to U.S. parents, they especially discourage negative emotional expression (Kojima 2000).

Socializers' tendencies to discuss emotions, if nested within a warm parent-child relationship, assist the child acquiring emotional competence (Kochanoff 2001). Parents directly teach their children about emotions, explaining its relation to an observed event or expression, directing attention to salient emotional cues, and helping children understand and manage their own responses.

Parents who are aware of emotions and talk about them in a differentiated manner (e.g., clarifying and explaining, rather than "preaching") assist their children in experiencing and regulating their own emotions. Children of such parents gradually formulate a coherent body of knowledge about emotional expressions, situations, and causes (Denham, Cook, and Zoller 1992; Denham, Zoller, and Couchoud 1994).

Late twentieth-century research suggests that Japanese mothers also talk to their preschoolers about emotions (e.g., Clancy, 1999; Sonoda and Muto 1996). They use emotion language for similar reasons as U.S. mothers; what differs is the content of their conversations, which focus on aspects of emotion relevant for Japanese culture.

Thus, positive elements of emotion socialization seem clear. Moreover, there is some evidence that parents' support of one another also helps to ensure such positive elements (Denham and Kochanoff, in press). However, do beneficial aspects of parents' socialization of emotion differ across children's ages, or across parents? Although more research is needed in this area, it is predicted that these socializing techniques would occur across development and parents, albeit with different emphasized emotions, and different aspects yielding positive child outcomes. In part, however, these questions require an elucidation of children's changing skills of emotional competence.

Expression and experience of emotions: An important element of emotional competence is emotional expressiveness, the sending of affective messages. Emotions must be expressed in keeping with the child's goals, and in accordance with the social context; goals of self and others must be coordinated. Thus, emotional competence includes *expressing emotions* in a way that is advantageous to moment-to-moment interaction and relationships over time (Halberstadt, Denham, and Dunsmore 2001).

First, emotionally competent individuals are aware that an affective message needs to be sent in a given context. But what affective message should be sent, for interaction to proceed smoothly? Children slowly learn which expressions of emotion facilitate specific goals. Second, children also come to determine the appropriate affective message, one that works in the setting or with a specific playmate. Third, children must also learn how to send the affective message convincingly. Method, intensity, and timing of an affective message are crucial to its meaning, and eventual success or failure.

After preschool, children learn that their goals are not always met by freely showing their most intense feelings. For example, grade-schoolers regulate anger in anticipation of the negative consequences they expect in specific situations or from specific persons (e.g., Zeman and Shipman 1996). Along with the *cool rule* mandating more muted emotions within most social settings, older children's emotional messages become more complex, with the use of more blended signals, and better differentiated expressions of social emotions.

These general tenets of competent experience and expression of emotion may be universal, but children from different cultures differ in the emotions they express. For example, Japanese preschoolers show less anger and distress in conflict situations than U.S. children, even though the two groups' prosocial and conflict *behaviours* do not differ (Zahn-Waxler et al. 1996). These differences fit the Japanese taboo on publicly displayed negative emotions.

Japanese toddlers and preschoolers' expressiveness is not always different from that of their U.S. peers'. For example, they express empathy in response to others' distress. Even this similarity, however, may arise from differing cultural imperatives. Japanese youngsters are encouraged to feel as one with their group, whereas Western children are encouraged to feel the state of another as part of their increasingly autonomous regulation of emotional states. The import of these subtle differences needs further exploration.

Understanding Emotions: Emotion knowledge predicts later social functioning, such as social acceptance by peers. By preschool, most children can infer basic emotions from expressions or situations, and understand their consequences. Preschoolers gradually come to differentiate among the negative emotions, and become increasingly capable of using emotional language. Furthermore, young children begin to identify other peoples' emotions, even when they may differ from their own (Denham, 1986; Fabes et al. 1988; Fabes et al. 1991).

Grade-schoolers become more aware of emotional experience, including multiple emotions, and realize that inner and outer emotional states may differ. By middle school, children comprehend the time course of emotions, display rules associated with emotional situations, and moral emotions. They now have an adult-like sense of how different events elicit different emotions in different people, and that enduring personality traits may impact individualized emotional reactions (Gnepp 1989; Olthof, Ferguson, and Luiten 1989).

These general tenets of competent emotion knowledge seem similar for Japanese children. For example, even two-year-olds use some emotion language; by the end of preschool, their understanding of culturally appropriate emotion language is acute (Clancy 1999; Matsuo 1997). They begin to understand dissemblance of emotion (Sawada 1997). As in U.S. research, however, there is a relative dearth of research on older children.

Emotion Regulation: Emotion regulation is necessary when the presence or absence of emotional expression and experience interferes with a person's goals. Negative or positive emotions can need regulating, when they threaten to overwhelm or need to be amplified. Children learn to retain or enhance those emotions that are relevant and helpful, to attenuate those that are relevant but not helpful, and to dampen those that are irrelevant. These skills help them to experience a greater sense of well-being and maintain satisfying relationships with others (Thompson 1994).

Early in preschool, much of this emotion regulation is biobehavioral (e.g., thumb sucking), and much is supported by adults. Important cognitive foundations of emotion regulation contribute to the developmental changes observed in emotional competence from preschool to adolescence. Preschoolers gradually begin to use independent coping strategies for emotion regulation, and grade-schoolers refine these strategies—problemsolving, support-seeking, distancing, internalizing, externalizing, distraction, reframing/redefining, cognitive "blunting" (i.e., convincing oneself that one's distress is minimal), and denial.

Older children are uniquely aware of the multiple strategies at their command, and know which are adaptive in specific situations. They also use more cognitive and problem-solving, and fewer support-seeking, strategies. Adolescents appraise the controllability of emotional experiences, shift thoughts intentionally, and reframe situations to reach new solutions (Saarni 1997).

Japanese children, as noted above, are initially very close to their mothers, who assist them in emotion regulation even more than Western mothers. Some researchers have noted, however, that once emotionally distressed, Japanese children find it harder to regain their equilibrium (Kojima 2000). It could be that extended maternal coregulation, coupled with stricter cultural display rules, make it more difficult for these children to self-regulate once distressed. More research is needed to follow up on these findings.

Emotional Control and Maturity

Controlling your emotion begins with a deliberate decision to keep composure and emotional retrain at all times. You should be very mindful of your feelings in every situation whether it is exuberant or sorrowful. You should avoid the belief that people are entitled to loose control in special occasions or that people have the right to let out their emotions in specific circumstances. You should stop adhering to the belief that "people are just humans" because what makes people humans is their ability to tame their desires and emotions.

You should understand that emotion is actually dependent on your behaviour and not the other way around. To put it simply, you feel sad because you realize that you are frowning, contrary to the popular notion that you frown because you realize that you are sad. In social psychology, it has been discovered behaviour influences emotions, and not the other way around. With this key information at hand, you are empowered with the ability to influence feelings by modifying behaviour.

A common cause of emotional outbursts is having problems. Oftentimes, when people are faced with difficulties, they react by panicking or by being angry. However, these are not solutions to the initial problem; they are sources of problems themselves. When you are in a state of panic or in a rage of anger, your mind is clouded with emotions that the situation is not seen clearly. This does make it harder to think of concrete solutions to the problem being dealt with. Whenever a problem comes, instead of immediately throwing tantrums or pacing restlessly, you should stop, breath, and evaluate the entirety of the circumstance. This way, the problem can be viewed in a clearer perspective, and solutions may be thought out more logically.

One very valuable tool in emotional control is the ability to pause. While there are no pause and play buttons in real life, people have the capability to stop themselves, and take a break in certain situations that usually cause emotional outbursts. Before shouting and screaming out of a disappointing occurrence, you should first take a break to think and reflect. Pausing in itself is a form of emotional control. At this point, you can think if letting go of the emotions is indeed necessary. You should also think of the consequences that the emotional explosion would entail. If the emotions involved in the situation are too strong to withhold, you can think of reasonable emotional expressions such as crying instead of screaming when you are depressed, or smiling instead of jumping around when you are elated.

The problem with most people who are unable to control their emotions is that they dwell too much on the present situation. It is undeniable that the height of emotions experienced in certain circumstances could be overwhelming. However, these are also the times when you are vulnerable to do things that you might regret later on. To avoid this, it is important to examine how things would go in the future. Emotional control is indeed difficult to master. But with will power and determination, it can be possibly achieved. You just have to be aware that emotions do not really have the power to overcome people. On the contrary, people have the ability to watch over their emotions and control them to what they think is necessary.

Place of Emotions in Life

An emotion is the meaning we give to our felt states of arousal. Psychologists consider emotions to be complex states involving diverse aspects. On the one hand an emotion is a physiological state of arousal; on the other, it also involves an object as having a certain significance or value to the individual. Emotions are dynamically fed by our drives and dispositions; they are also interlocked with other emotions, related to an individual's beliefs, a wide-ranging network of symbols and the "cultural ethos" of a society.

Emotions basically involve dispositions to act by way of approach or withdrawal. Let us take an example to illustrate this. A man who walks a long distance across a forest track feels thirsty, he is attracted by the sight of water in a passing stream and he approaches; but there is a fierce animal close to the stream and he is impelled to withdraw or fight; if he withdraws he might then have a general feeling of anxiety, and if he gets back home safely he will be relieved. Thus perception of objects and situations is followed by a kind of appraisal of them as attractive or harmful. These appraisals initiate tendencies to feel in a certain manner and an impulse to act in a desirable way. All states of appraisal do not initiate action; for instance, in joy we like a passive continuation of the existing state and in grief we generally give up hope. Though there may be certain biologically built-in patterns of expressing emotions, learning plays a key role. Learning influences both the type and intensity of arousal as well as the control and expression of emotions.

The emotional development of people has been the subject of serious study. There are significant differences in the emotional development of people depending on the relevant cultural and social variables. In fact, certain societies are prone to give prominence to certain types of emotions (a dominant social ethos). There are also differences regarding the degree of expressiveness and control of emotions. The important point is that each of us develops a relatively consistent pattern of emotional development, coloured by the individual's style of life.

Significance of Emotional Intelligence

Emotional Intelligence as an Approach to Teaching and Learning Processes

Concerning **emotional intelligence** I believe that we need to reassess our thinking as we do in the world in general. We cannot put too much emphasis on one narrow or limited feature but should consider a person as a whole. We need skilled people, professionals with scientific competence who can define what **emotional intelligence** is all about. In the past **intelligence** was defined in a limited way with emphasis on reading and arithmetic. Many other features were left in the background until their importance was also acknowledged. What kind of educational system will be developed in Finland depends on what kind of all-round **significance** is attached to it. I claim that all the big goals that Finland and Europe, for example, have concerning competitiveness, require a working educational system. It is no use talking about a competitive economy or society if it does not offer the kind of education that inspires and motivates people to work towards those goals. Education, on the other hand, is not only about economic competitiveness but also about contending with oneself and achieving one's moral goals. In this realm we don't seem to have a vision. Everywhere people are waiting to see what others do. I don't mean that we would need another Leonardo da Vinci or Immanuel Kant or some accomplished pedagogue who would give us answers. It is not the world of one great man or woman that I'm after but some kind of school of thought, a cultural trend or, in formal language, ideology to define what we are as people. If we get this kind of inspiration and realize that we exist and are inspired when our feelings are aroused, then we are talking about **emotional intelligence**. What is included is music and painting (not necessarily pompous music or imposing art), media and traditional theatre but also strong mathematical competence and capacity for abstract reasoning. All this is part of the Zeitgeist, the spirit of the age, which is our responsibility to create. If educational visionaries and school reformers cannot create this spirit, where else can it come from? An individual teacher or professor may do their best in their own work but if their efforts are wrecked by bureaucratic machinery, nothing will be reformed. This is why it is good to point out and emphasize that emotions can be the basis of all this change. Then we should consider what that entails.

Educational Programmes and Curricula from the Point of View of Emotional Intelligence

They are of more importance than has been generally acknowledged so far. When it comes to education and educational programmes, the goal can be a good life or a good and just world, which is a world of knowledge and understanding. Finding a good life, on the other hand, requires the ability to perceive **emotional** life and its **significance**. In fact I claim emotion can be an essential initiator in the birth of cognitive and traditional intellectual accomplishments. It is a source of motivation. The fact that a person becomes interested may be a sign of an ability to move in the realm of **emotional** life. What media researchers have always known and what has been taken into account in the media education of some countries, are the dimensions of cognitive, **emotional**, moral, aesthetic education and so on.

It is a recognized fact that in the media, emotions are created. As a counter reaction young people and people in general should be able to perceive that emotions are being created *for* them, emotions whose origin is not in them. It is not bad in itself because when actors fall in love in a film, it can have a positive effect on the viewers. What is more important, however, is that people would fall in love in real life, too, and not only through films. In other words, I claim that to induce enthusiasm, motivation and persistent positive intellectual curiosity we need to be aware of **emotional** life and include it in the preparation of curricula.

Examples of Taking Emotional Life into Consideration

I don't actually know of any existing programme which does this because I work in research which is not very close to the operational level. However, I can take an example of the international work that I am involved in, which perhaps shows how **emotional** life could be taken into account. I studied the life and work of Anton Chekhov in Taganrog in the southwest of Russia. His attitude to knowledge and technology was very positive and balanced because he also wanted to preserve nature and values instead of letting technology and knowledge change life too much. He was talking to a young lawyer about something when he suddenly, in the middle of the conversation, asked the young man if he liked the gramophone, which at that time was a new invention.

The young man answered that he did. Chekhov said that *he* didn't. When the young man wondered why not, Chekhov replied that it did have moving sound and music but it was somehow dead, it was empty, it did not have emotions. Then they continued their conversation about photography and other things. This conversation crystallizes the concrete situation Chekhov lived in a hundred years ago and which is present in today's teaching situations. Young people have mechanical devices for reproducing art and music. Day in day out they wear their headphones. However, a machine is always a machine. No matter how interactive it is, it is devoid of all the sensitivity that is involved when you are making music in real life. A machine cannot identify the elements of the situation. If this is lacking, interaction between people is on a mechanical level. There is a difference between listening to a perfect CD and being at a live concert where one single cough is an expression of the tension in the air, let alone the actual singing and playing. The different elements of the situation regarding speed, tempo, emphasis or anything else that cannot be repeated are essential in the situation. They touch emotion. Emotion is involved. The same applies to speech. A person may speak well and learn mechanically to use good structures and express himself well, yet disregard the social situation. Without any other concrete example I claim that in order to be able to consider **emotional intelligence** sensibly, it has to be done in situational contexts. Of course the intellectual and background elements are also needed but it is only in the immediate social context that the emotions come into play.

Emotional Intelligence in the Co-operation between Schools and Homes

Co-operation between schools and homes must involve a sense of community but I don't think we can emphasize and use only this. I speak again from the ivory tower of university life because I am in no contact with the interaction between schools and homes in today's society other than through my grandchildren. But I am under the impression that many people are clueless about parenthood, at least when considered from the point of view of my generation.

Nowadays both parents pursue their own career and the home is different from what it was a few decades ago when schools were built and current educational thinking was developed. Nowadays responsibility is too easily shifted from homes on to institutions, such as schools, kindergartens, day-care centres and clubs. A prerequisite for a good life and well-being is that there are emotions and that they can be reciprocated. If there are no emotions in a home, it is impossible to develop them from the outside. Now I speak as an amateur with no factual knowledge of the matter but I would like to claim that *caring as a way of thinking* or a world where parents are made sensitive to what is happening in the world of children would be good. Whether something like that exists or not I have no way of knowing.

Moral Development

Impacting Moral and Character Development

Campbell and Bond (1982) state there are four major questions to be addressed when focusing on character development:

1. what is good character;
2. what causes or prevents it;

3. how can it be measured so that efforts at improvement can have corrective feedback;and
4. how can it best be developed?

As previously discussed, good character is defined in terms of one's actions. Character development traditionally has focused on those traits or values appropriate for the industrial age such as obedience to authority, work ethic, working in group under supervision, etc. However, as discussed in the SCANS report (1991) and Huitt's (1997) critique, modern education must promote character based on values appropriate for the information age: truthfulness, honesty, integrity, individual responsibility, humility, wisdom, justice, steadfastness, dependability, etc.

In terms of what influences character development, Campbell and Bond (1982) propose the following as major factors in the moral development and behaviour of youth in contemporary America:

1. heredity
2. early childhood experience
3. Modelling by important adults and older youth
4. peer influence
5. the general physical and social environment
6. the communications media
7. what is taught in the schools and other institutions
8. specific situations and roles that elicit corresponding behaviour.

These sources of influence are listed in approximate order of least tractable to most tractable in order to suggest why we often seek solutions to social problems through schools. It is important to realize that while schools do and should play a role in the development of character, families, communities, and society in general also have an important influence (Huitt, 1999).

The measurement of character has proven difficult since character, by definition, involves behaviour, but character is often defined in terms of traits (i.e., honesty, integrity, etc.).

Some possible measures suggested by Campbell and Bond (1982) are:

1. student discipline;
2. student suicide rates;
3. crimes: assault, burglary, homicides;
4. pregnancy rates of teenage girls; and
5. prosocial activities.

Bennett (1993) proposed a list of cultural indicators that he believes could be used as measures of the character of our society. In addition, he cited a number of social trends that he believes have impacted these indicators. The following table provides an overview of how these have changed from 1960 to 1990.

Earlier Theoretical Models: Psychoanalysis and Behaviourism

Theories have approached morality differently. Sigmund Freud (1856–1939) described *Oedipus complex* to explain the origins of moral conscience, called the *superego.* The Oedipus complex occurs when a child loves the opposite sex parent and, in order to avoid the anxiety and fear of punishment that this causes, the child identifies with the same sex parent. The child incorporates the same sex parent's prohibitions, starting with "Do not love (sexually) your parent."

For behaviourist theorists, such as Robert R. Sears, Robert Grinder, and Albert Bandura (1982), conscience or morality was considered analogous to the phenomenon of resistance to extinction. H. Hartshorne and M. A. May, at the end of the 1920s, were pioneers in this line of research. Later, Robert Sears, Eleanor Maccoby, and Harry Levin (1957) and other researchers studied the influence of maternal and paternal disciplines upon development of the conscience.

These studies found that warm and affectionate parents, who reason with their children rather than punish them physically, are more successful in having their children assimilate the moral values of the culture. Cognitive behaviourists have added other dimensions to this process, such as *expectancies* (what the child expects is going to happen), *incentive value* (how much the child wants something), *hypothesis testing* ("If I do this, then that will happen"), and *self-efficacy* (one's capacity and confidence on doing something) (Bandura 1977, 1978). In the psychoanalytic and behaviourist models, morality seems to be something that comes from outside, from society, which is internalized.

Theories of Moral Development

Evaluating theories of moral development is difficult due to lack of a consistent definition. For some, moral development is seen principally as ability to reason about universal principles of justice and fairness (moral judgment). For others, it is a matter of ability to empathize with and act to alleviate others' suffering (compassion). Both reasoning and compassion are necessary in formulating moral actions; however, it is the relative importance of each that distinguishes different theories.

Two of the main modern theories of moral development, Kohlberg's (1984) and Gilligan's (1982), are based on long standing, underlying philosophical arguments about the basis of moral development. Each is a stage theory in which people develop from one stage to the next as they grow in ability to make complex judgments. Where the theories differ is on how people make judgments.

Kohlberg's (1984) theory focuses more on the use of reason to draw conclusions about what ought to be done to achieve justice and fairness in a particular situation. Altruism, compassion and empathy are less important than principles of justice, and are not the main part of the reasoned process of coming to moral decisions. The moral reasoner is one who knows that a moral decision is required, understands that principles need to be applied universally, thinks of the greatest good for the most people, and then makes a decision based on abstract principles of justice and fairness. Kohlberg's theory follows Piaget's and Inhelder's (1969) thinking about the stages of mental development. Because Kohlberg's (1984) theory is based on the ability to reason abstractly, young children are not seen as being able to reason about moral issues yet; they are pre-moral. Another major avenue of exploration of moral issues is based on altruism. Modern philosophers such as Blum (1987) and Matthews (1994) suggested that childhood responsiveness to others is a primary moral characteristic. Responsiveness requires both a cognitive and affective grasp of a situation. It does not require true empathy yet, nor does it require that children be aware of why they act as they do, only that the act has been done. What is required for an act to be moral is a recognition of the emotions of the other, and of the action needed to change the situation. What changes from childhood to adulthood is the amount and type of experience the person brings to the situation. For example, the adult might offer advice the young child might not yet know about. This model of morality has some similarity to the model of care developed by Gilligan (1982). In Gilligan's model it is the interrelationships among people that are important, and these are based on empathic responses between people. Responding to another's pain or difficulty is the basis of moral action. This requires an empathic attitude to others, a sensitivity to others' needs, and a wish to act with these needs in mind. This type of thinking reflects sensitivity towards others rather than a focus on reasoning about what is a principled or unprincipled act.

While Kohlberg's (1984) theory has been directly tested with gifted children, especially through use of the Defining Issues Test (Rest, 1979), there has been little direct application of Gilligan's (1982) theory to the gifted. Like many other researchers, Gilligan appears to use some data from gifted children, but does not distinguish between data obtained from gifted children and more average subjects. For example, an extensive study at the Emma Willard School illustrated the moral decisions made in the context of relationships with other girls (Gilligan, Lyons, & Hanmer, 1989). Many of the girls described appear to be quite gifted.

A third approach was suggested by Dabrowski whose work has been described and interpreted by Piechowski (1986; 1991). Dabrowski specifically studied gifted youth and adults and developed a theory of emotional development that was based on observations of his gifted subjects. Piechowski (1991), in interpreting the theory, noted that gifted youth, like gifted adults, feel a deep longing for ideals in life, such as justice, fairness, honesty, and responsibility. Gifted children also expect that adults ought to be able to do something to right the wrongs of the world and may be profoundly disappointed by their lack of doing so.

Dabrowski's theory (Piechowski, 1986) does not specifically discuss young gifted children. Dabrowski focused on adolescents and adults; thus, his theory required both life experience and ability to evaluate concepts in order for people to develop further in emotional and moral complexity. Like the theories of Kohlberg (1984) and Gilligan (1982), Dabrowski's theory suggests stages of development (five), with growth towards an ideal of self-actualization in the final stage, realized by few. For young gifted children, the applicability of Dabrowski's theory lies in his description of exceptional emotional sensitivity and intensity that can accompany giftedness. As the child grows into adolescence and identity is formed through evaluation of personal values, the person may develop through Dabrowski's stages. Piechowski (1991) described a number of adolescents who appeared to show potential for the kind of inner growth in both emotional self-awareness and moral sensitivity described by Dabrowski's theory. For these adolescents, the development of self is accompanied throughout life by growth in moral sensitivity, integration of universal concepts of justice and fairness and universal compassion.

Piaget's and Kohlberg's Stages of Moral Development

Piaget's Stages of Moral Development

Piaget studied many aspects of moral judgment, but most of his findings fit into a two-stage theory. Children younger than 10 or 11 years think about moral dilemmas one way; older children consider them differently. As we have seen, younger children regard rules as fixed and absolute. They believe that rules are handed down by adults or by God and that one cannot change them. The older child's view is more relativistic. He or she understands that it is permissible to change rules if everyone agrees. Rules are not sacred and absolute but are devices which humans use to get along cooperatively.

At approximately the same time—10 or 11 years—children's moral thinking undergoes other shifts. In particular, younger children base their moral judgments more on consequences, whereas older children base their judgments on intentions. When, for example, the young child hears about one boy who broke 15 cups trying to help his mother and another boy who broke only one cup trying to steal cookies, the young child thinks that the first boy did worse. The child primarily considers the amount of damage—the consequences—whereas the older child is more likely to judge wrongness in terms of the motives underlying the act (Piaget, 1932, p. 137).

There are many more details to Piaget's work on moral judgment, but he essentially found a series of changes that occur between the ages of 10 and 12, just when the child begins to enter the general stage of formal operations.

Intellectual development, however, does not stop at this point. This is just the beginning of formal operations, which continue to develop at least until age 16. Accordingly, one might expect thinking about moral issues to continue to develop throughout adolescence. Kohlberg therefore interviewed both children and adolescents about moral dilemmas, and he did find stages that go well beyond Piaget's. He uncovered six stages, only the first three of which share many features with Piaget's stages.

Kohlberg's Stages of Moral Development

Lawrence Kohlberg's stages of moral development constitute an adaptation of a psychological theory originally conceived of by the Swiss psychologist Jean Piaget. Kohlberg, while a psychology postgraduate student at the University of Chicago expanded and developed throughout the course of his life.

The theory holds that moral reasoning, the basis for ethical behaviour, has six identifiable developmental stages, each more adequate at responding to moral dilemmas than its predecessor. Kohlberg followed the development of moral judgment far beyond the ages studied earlier by Piaget, who also claimed that logic and morality develop through constructive stages. Expanding on Piaget's work, Kohlberg determined that the process of moral development was principally concerned with justice, and that it continued throughout the individual's lifetime, a notion that spawned dialogue on the philosophical implications of such research.

Kohlberg relied for his studies on stories such as the Heinz dilemma, and was interested in how individuals would justify their actions if placed in similar moral dilemmas. He then analyzed the form of moral reasoning displayed, rather than its conclusion, and classified it as belonging to one of six distinct stages.

There have been critiques of the theory from several perspectives. Some argue that it emphasizes justice to the exclusion of other moral values, such as caring; or that there is such an overlap between stages that they should more properly be regarded as separate domains; or that evaluations of the reasons for moral choices are mostly *post hoc* rationalizations (by both decision makers and psychologists studying them) of essentially intuitive decisions.

Nevertheless, an entirely new field within psychology was created as a result of Kohlberg's theory, and according to Haggbloom et al.'s study of the most eminent psychologists of the 20th century, Kohlberg was the 16th most frequently cited psychologist in introductory psychology textbooks throughout the century, as well as the 30th most eminent overall.

Stages

Kohlberg's six stages can be more generally grouped into three levels of two stages each: pre-conventional, conventional and post-conventional. Following Piaget's constructivist requirements for a stage model, as described in his theory of cognitive development, it is extremely rare to regress backward in stages—to lose the use of higher stage abilities. Stages cannot be skipped; each provides a new and necessary perspective, more comprehensive and differentiated than its predecessors but integrated with them.

Level 1 (Pre-Conventional)

1. Obedience and punishment orientation
   (*How can I avoid punishment?*)
2. Self-interest orientation
   (*What's in it for me?*)

Level 2 (Conventional)

3. Interpersonal accord and conformity
   (*Social norms*)
   (*The good boy/good girl attitude*)
4. Authority and social-order maintaining orientation
   (*Law and order morality*)

Level 3 (Post-Conventional)

5. Social contract orientation
6. Universal ethical principles
   (*Principled conscience*).

Pre-Conventional

The pre-conventional level of moral reasoning is especially common in children, although adults can also exhibit this level of reasoning. Reasoners at this level judge the morality of an action by its direct consequences. The pre-conventional level consists of the first and second stages of moral development, and is solely concerned with the self in an egocentric manner.

In **Stage one** (obedience and punishment driven), individuals focus on the direct consequences of their actions on themselves. For example, an action is perceived as morally wrong if the perpetrator is punished. "The last time I did that I got spanked so I will not do it again." The worse the punishment for the act is, the more "bad" the act is perceived to be. This can give rise to an inference that even innocent victims are guilty in proportion to their suffering. It is "egocentric", lacking recognition that others' points of view are different from one's own. There is "deference to superior power or prestige".

Stage two (self-interest driven) espouses the "what's in it for me" position, in which right behaviour is defined by whatever is in the individual's best interest. Stage two reasoning shows a limited interest in the needs of others, but only to a point where it might further the individual's own interests. As a result, concern for others is not based on loyalty or intrinsic respect, but rather a "you scratch my back, and I'll scratch yours" mentality. The lack of a societal perspective in the pre-conventional level is quite different from the social contract (stage five), as all actions have the purpose of serving the individual's own needs or interests. For the stage two theorist, the world's perspective is often seen as morally relative.

Conventional

The conventional level of moral reasoning is typical of adolescents and adults. Those who reason in a conventional way judge the morality of actions by comparing them to society's views and expectations. The conventional level consists of the third and fourth stages of moral development.

In **Stage three** (interpersonal accord and conformity driven), the self enters society by filling social roles. Individuals are receptive to approval or disapproval from others as it reflects society's accordance with the perceived role. They try to be a "good boy" or "good girl" to live up to these expectations, having learned that there is inherent value in doing so. Stage three reasoning may judge the morality of an action by evaluating its consequences in terms of a person's relationships, which now begin to include things like respect, gratitude and the "golden rule". "I want to be liked and thought well of; apparently, not being naughty makes people like me." Desire to maintain rules and authority exists only to further support these social roles. The intentions of actions play a more significant role in reasoning at this stage; "they mean well ...".

In **Stage four** (authority and social order obedience driven), it is important to obey laws, dictums and social conventions because of their importance in maintaining a functioning society. Moral reasoning in stage four is thus beyond the need for individual approval exhibited in stage three; society must learn to transcend individual needs. A central ideal or ideals often prescribe what is right and wrong, such as in the case of fundamentalism. If one person violates a law, perhaps everyone would—thus there is an obligation and a duty to uphold laws and rules. When someone does violate a law, it is morally wrong; culpability is thus a significant factor in this stage as it separates the bad domains from the good ones. Most active members of society remain at stage four, where morality is still predominantly dictated by an outside force.

Post-Conventional

The post-conventional level, also known as the principled level, consists of stages five and six of moral development. There is a growing realization that individuals are separate entities from society, and that the individual's own perspective may take precedence over society's view. Because of this level's "nature of self before others", the behaviour of post-conventional individuals, especially those at stage 6, can be confused with that of those at the pre-conventional level.

In **Stage five** (social contract driven), individuals are viewed as holding different opinions and values. Similarly, laws are regarded as social contracts rather than rigid dictums. Those which do not promote the general welfare should be changed when necessary to meet "the greatest good for the greatest number of people". This is achieved through majority decision, and inevitable compromise. Thus democratic government is ostensibly based on stage five reasoning.

In **Stage six** (universal ethical principles driven), moral reasoning is based on abstract reasoning using universal ethical principles. Laws are valid only insofar as they are grounded in justice, and a commitment to justice carries with it an obligation to disobey unjust laws. Rights are unnecessary, as social contracts are not essential for deontic moral action. Decisions are not reached hypothetically in a conditional way but rather categorically in an absolute way, as in the philosophy of Immanuel Kant. This involves an individual imagining what they would do in another's shoes, if they believed what that other person imagines to be true. The resulting consensus is the action taken. In this way action is never a means but always an end in itself; the individual acts because it is right, and not because it is instrumental, expected, legal, or previously agreed upon. Although Kohlberg insisted that stage six exists, he found it difficult to identify individuals who consistently operated at that level.

Further Stages

In his empirical studies of individuals throughout their life Kohlberg observed that some had apparently undergone moral stage regression. Faced with the option of either conceding that moral regression could occur or revising his theory, Kohlberg chose the latter, postulating the existence of sub-stages in which the emerging stage has not yet been fully integrated into the personality. In particular Kohlberg noted a stage 4½ or 4+, a transition from stage four to stage five, that shared characteristics of both. In this stage the individual is disaffected with the arbitrary nature of law and order reasoning; culpability is frequently turned from being defined by society to viewing society itself as culpable. This stage is often mistaken for the moral relativism of stage two, as the individual views those interests of society which conflict with their own as being relatively and morally wrong. Kohlberg noted that this was often observed in students entering college.

Kohlberg suggested that there may a seventh stage—Transcendental Morality, or Morality of Cosmic Orientation—which linked religion with moral reasoning. Kohlberg's difficulties in obtaining empirical evidence for even a sixth stage, however, led him to emphasize the speculative nature of his seventh stage.

Unit-V

Learning

Nature and Importance of Learning

Learning is acquiring new knowledge, behaviours, skills, values, preferences or understanding, and may involve synthesizing different types of information. The ability to learn is possessed by humans, animals and some machines. Progress over time tends to follow learning curves.

Human learning may occur as part of education or personal development. It may be goal-oriented and may be aided by motivation. The study of how learning occurs is part of neuropsychology, educational psychology, learning theory, and pedagogy

Learning may occur as a result of habituation or classical conditioning, seen in many animal species, or as a result of more complex activities such as play, seen only in relatively intelligent animals and humans. Learning may occur consciously or without conscious awareness. There is evidence for human Behavioural learning prenatally, in which habituation has been observed as early as 32 weeks into gestation, indicating that the central nervous system is sufficiently developed and primed for learning and memory to occur very early on in development.

Play has been approached by several theorists as the first form of learning. Children play, experiment with the world, learn the rules, and learn to interact. Vygotsky supports that play is pivotal for children's development, since they make meaning of their environment through play.

Individual Differences in Learning

Simple Non-associative Learning

Habituation: In psychology, habituation is an example of non-associative learning in which there is a progressive diminution of Behavioural response probability with repetition of a stimulus. It is another form of integration. An animal first responds to a stimulus, but if it is neither rewarding nor harmful the animal reduces subsequent responses. One example of this can be seen in small song birds-if a stuffed owl (or similar predator) is put into the cage, the birds initially react to it as though it were a real predator. Soon the birds react less, showing habituation. If another stuffed owl is introduced (or the same one removed and re-introduced), the birds react to it again as though it were a predator, demonstrating that it is only a very specific stimulus that is habituated to (namely, one particular unmoving owl in one place). Habituation has been shown in essentially every species of animal, including the large protozoan *Stentor Coeruleus*.

Sensitization: Sensitization is an example of non-associative learning in which the progressive amplification of a response follows repeated administrations of a stimulus (Bell et al., 1995). An everyday example of this mechanism is the repeated tonic stimulation of peripheral nerves that will occur if a person rubs his arm continuously. After a while, this stimulation will create a warm sensation that will eventually turn painful. The pain is the result of the progressively amplified synaptic response of the peripheral nerves warning the person that the stimulation is harmful. Sensitization is thought to underlie both adaptive as well as maladaptive learning processes in the organism.

Associative Learning

Associative learning is the process by which an element is learned through association with a separate, pre-occurring element.

Operant Conditioning

Operant conditioning is the use of consequences to modify the occurrence and form of behaviour. *Operant conditioning* is distinguished from Pavlovian conditioning in that operant conditioning deals with the modification of voluntary behaviour. Discrimination learning is a major form of operant conditioning. One form of it is called Errorless learning.

Classical Conditioning

The typical paradigm for classical conditioning involves repeatedly pairing an unconditioned stimulus (which unfailingly evokes a particular response) with another previously neutral stimulus (which does not normally evoke the response). Following conditioning, the response occurs both to the unconditioned stimulus and to the other, unrelated stimulus (now referred to as the "conditioned stimulus"). The response to the conditioned stimulus is termed a *conditioned response*.

Imprinting

Imprinting is the term used in psychology and ethology to describe any kind of phase-sensitive learning (learning occurring at a particular age or a particular life stage) that is rapid and apparently independent of the consequences of behaviour. It was first used to describe situations in which an animal or person learns the characteristics of some stimulus, which is therefore said to be "imprinted" onto the subject.

Observational Learning

The most common human learning process is imitation; one's personal repetition of an observed behaviour, such as a dance. Humans can copy three types of information simultaneously: the demonstrator's goals, actions and environmental outcomes. Through copying these types of information, (most) infants will tune into their surrounding culture.

Play

Play generally describes behaviour which has no particular end in itself, but improves performance in similar situations in the future. This is seen in a wide variety of vertebrates besides humans, but is mostly limited to mammals and birds. Cats are known to play with a ball of string when young, which gives them experience with catching prey. Besides inanimate objects, animals may play with other members of their own species or other animals, such as orcas playing with seals they have caught.

Play involves a significant cost to animals, such as increased vulnerability to predators and the risk of injury and possibly infection. It also consumes energy, so there must be significant benefits associated with play for it to have evolved. Play is generally seen in younger animals, suggesting a link with learning. However, it may also have other benefits not associated directly with learning, for example improving physical fitness.

Enculturation

Enculturation is the process by which a person learns the requirements of the culture by which he or she is surrounded, and acquires values and behaviours that are appropriate or necessary in that culture. The influences which as part of this process limit, direct or shape the individual, whether deliberately of not, include parents, other adults, and peers. If successful, enculturation results in competence in the language, values and rituals of the culture.

Multimedia Learning

The learning where learner uses multimedia learning environments (Mayer, 2001). This type of learning relies on dual-coding theory (Paivio, 1971).

e-Learning and Augmented Learning

Electronic learning or e-learning is a general term used to refer to Internet-based networked computer-enhanced learning. A specific and always more diffused e-learning is mobile learning (m-Learning), it uses different mobile telecommunication equipments, such as cellular phones.

When a learner interacts with the e-learning environment, it's called augmented learning. By adapting to the needs of individuals, the context-driven instruction can be dynamically tailored to the learner's natural environment. Augmented digital content may include text, images, video, audio (music and voice). By personalizing instruction, augmented learning has been shown to improve learning performance for a lifetime.

Rote Learning

Rote learning is a technique which avoids understanding the inner complexities and inferences of the subject that is being learned and instead focuses on memorizing the material so that it can be recalled by the learner exactly the way it was read or heard. The major practice involved in rote learning techniques is *learning by repetition*, based on the idea that one will be able to quickly recall the meaning of the material the more it is repeated. Rote learning is used in diverse areas, from mathematics to music to religion. Although it has been criticized by some schools of thought, rote learning is a necessity in many situations.

Informal Learning

Informal learning occurs through the experience of day-to-day situations (for example, one would learn to look ahead while walking because of the danger inherent in not paying attention to where one is going). It is learning from life, during a meal at table with parents, Play, exploring.

Formal Learning

Formal learning is learning that takes place within a teacher-student relationship, such as in a school system.

Nonformal Learning

Nonformal learning is organized learning outside the formal learning system. For example: learning by coming together with people with similar interests and exchanging viewpoints, in clubs or in (international) youth organizations, workshops.

Non-formal Learning and Combined Approaches

The educational system may use a combination of formal, informal, and non-formal learning methods. The UN and EU recognize these different forms of learning (cf. links below). In some schools students can get points that count in the formal-learning systems if they get work done in informal-learning circuits. They may be given time to assist international youth workshops and training courses, on the condition they prepare, contribute, share and can proof this offered valuable new insights, helped to acquire new skills, a place to get experience in organizing, teaching, etc.

In order to learn a skill, such as solving a Rubik's cube quickly, several factors come into play at once:

- Directions help one learn the patterns of solving a Rubik's cube
- Practicing the moves repeatedly and for extended time helps with "muscle memory" and therefore speed
- Thinking critically about moves helps find shortcuts, which in turn helps to speed up future attempts.
- The Rubik's cube's six colours help anchor solving it within the head.
- Occasionally revisiting the cube helps prevent negative learning or loss of skill.

Tangential Learning

Tangential Learning is the process by which some portion of people will self-educate if a topic is exposed to them in something that they already enjoy.

Dialogic Learning

Dialogic learning is the type of learning based on dialogue. Its conception is based on contributions of diverse disciplines.

Learning Factors in Emotion

Emotions may also be learned. For example, fear may be learned through **conditioning**, and once fear is learned, the drive to avoid it is a powerful motivator. The learning of some fears, however, as well as certain other emotions, may involve other processes, which are discussed later.

Emotional responses may be learned also through **Modelling.** The high incidence of violence in our society is seen by some to be related to the high incidence of violence in the media, particularly television and movies.

Learning Curves

The term learning curve refers to a graphical representation of the "average" rate of learning for an activity or tool. It can represent at a glance the initial difficulty of learning something and, to an extent, how much there is to learn after initial familiarity. For example, the Windows program Notepad is extremely simple to learn, but offers little after this. On the other extreme is the UNIX terminal editor vi, which is difficult to learn, but offers a wide array of features to master after the user has figured out how to work it. It is possible for something to be easy to learn, but difficult to master or hard to learn with little beyond this.

Initially introduced in educational and behavioural psychology, the term has acquired a broader interpretation over time, and expressions such as "experience curve", "improvement curve", "cost improvement curve", "progress curve", "progress function", "startup curve", and "efficiency curve" are often used interchangeably. In economics the subject is rates of "development", as development refers to a whole system learning process with varying rates of progression. Generally speaking all learning displays incremental change over time, but describes an "S" curve which has different appearances depending on the time scale of observation. It has now also become associated with the evolutionary theory of punctuated equilibrium and other kinds of revolutionary change in complex systems generally, relating to innovation, organization behaviour and the management of group learning, among other fields. These processes of rapidly emerging new form appear to take place by complex learning within the systems themselves, which when observable, display curves of changing rates that accelerate and decelerate.

The first person to describe the learning curve was Hermann Ebbinghaus in 1885. He found that the time required to memorize a nonsense syllable increased sharply as the number of syllables increased. Psychologist, Arthur Bills gave a more detailed description of learning curves in 1934. He also discussed the properties of different types of learning curves, such as negative acceleration, positive acceleration, plateaus, and ogive curves. In 1936, Theodore Paul Wright described the effect of learning on labour productivity in the aircraft industry and proposed a mathematical model of the learning curve.

The economic learning of productivity and efficiency generally follows the same kinds of experience curves and have interesting secondary effects. Efficiency and productivity improvement can be considered as whole organization or industry or economy learning processes, as well as for individuals. The general pattern is of first speeding up and then slowing down, as the practically achievable level of methodology improvement is reached. The effect of reducing local effort and resource use by learning improved methods paradoxically often has the opposite latent effect on the next larger scale system, by facilitating it's expansion, or Economic growth, as discussed in Jevon's paradox in the 1880s and updated in the Khazzoom-Brookes Postulate in the 1980s. That it means that the effect of saving energy may generally be to increase energy use has not yet been widely appreciated in the sustainability or global warming discussions.

Factors Influencing the Learning

Learning is not all about gaining something by the teachers or trainings but it can be the things that we learn from our everyday life experiences. It is better to learn from others experiences then to tolerate tough things yourself. Learning is not a single step process. It takes by and by processes to shape itself. Learning something is like keeping it in mind forever, it is not like remembering but to considering it the way it is and the way it can be.

There are many factors which have direct and indirect impacts upon the process of learning. They may be internal or external, attitudinal or aptitude concerned, physiological or histological, general or specific, environmental or non-environmental, social or non-social, professional or personal. It is up to the interaction of a person to the things around him/her. Environmental factors can be of various types like a person's daily routine, activities, people around him/her, etc. Non-environmental can be the general factors that are not concerned with the environs around a person. Physiological ones are like his/her functions that he/she uses to perform in his/her daily life. Histological are all about his/her outlook and expressions that make him/her to look like what he/she is. Internal ones are all about his/her internal thoughts and way of behaviours that he/she has to hide or show at times before others. External ones are all those factors which are to be imposed on him/her from outside milieus. Attitude is about the way he shows himself to others and it is the way of his/her behaviour. Aptitude is about his talent and ability to display him and to absorb things. Social factors are the factors which are impacting on him from the prevailing society. Non-social are all of the factors excluded from the social factors category. Professional are all those which are career concerned. Personal ones have the concern with private affairs of a person.

All of the factors if treating in positive manner will give an impetus to the learning process of individuals while have a negative impact on learning process if acting in a negative manner.

Theories of Learning: Conditioning, Classical and Operant (Pavlov, Skinner); Trial and Error (Thorndike)

Learning can be defined as the process leading to relatively permanent Behavioural change or potential Behavioural change. In other words, as we learn, we alter the way we perceive our environment, the way we interpret the incoming stimuli, and therefore the way we interact, or behave. John B. Watson (1878-1958) was the first to study how the process of learning affects our behaviour, and he formed the school of thought known as *Behaviourism*. The central idea behind behaviourism is that only observable behaviours are worthy of research since other abstraction such as a person's mood or thoughts are too subjective. This belief was dominant in psychological research in the United Stated for a good 50 years.

Perhaps the most well known Behaviourist is B. F. Skinner (1904-1990). Skinner followed much of Watson's research and findings, but believed that internal states could influence behaviour just as external stimuli. He is considered to be a *Radical Behaviourist* because of this belief, although nowadays it is believed that both internal and external stimuli influence our behaviour.

Behavioural Psychology is basically interested in how our behaviour results from the stimuli both in the environment and within ourselves. They study, often in minute detail, the behaviours we exhibit while controlling for as many other variables as possible. Often a grueling process, but results have helped us learn a great deal about our behaviours, the effect our environment has on us, how we learn new behaviours, and what motivates us to change or remain the same.

The 4 Factors That Form The Definition of Learning:

1) learning is inferred from a change in behaviour/ performance*
2) learning results in an inferred change in memory
3) learning is the result of experience
4) learning is relatively permanent.

This means that behaviour changes that are temporary or due to things like drugs, alcohol, etc., are not "learned".

*Behaviour Potential-once something is learned, an organism can exhibit a behaviour that indicates learning as occurred. Thus, once a behaviour has been "learned", it can be exhibited by "performance" of a corresponding behaviour.

It is the combination of these 4 factors that make our definition of learning. Or, you can go with a slightly less comprehensive definition that is offered in many text books: **Learning is a relatively durable change in behaviour or knowledge that is due to experience.**

We are going to discuss the two main types of learning examined by researchers, classical conditioning and operant conditioning.

I. Classical Conditioning

Classical Conditioning can be defined as a type of learning in which a stimulus acquires the capacity to evoke a **reflexive** response that was originally evoked by a different stimulus.

A. Ivan Pavlov-Russian physiologist interested in behaviour (digestion).

1) Pavlov was studying salivation in dogs-he was measuring the amount of salivation produced by the salivary glands of dogs by presenting them meat powder through a food dispenser.

   The dispenser would deliver the meat powder to which the animals salivated. However, what Pavlov noticed was that the food dispenser made a sound when delivering the powder, and that the dogs salivated before the powder was delivered. He realized that the dogs associated the sound (which occurred seconds before the powder actually arrived) with the delivery of the food. Thus, the dogs had "learned" that when the sound occurred, the meat powder was going to arrive.

   This is conditioning (Stimulus-Response; S-R Bonds). The stimulus (sound of food dispenser) produced a response (salivation). It is important to note that at this point, we are talking about reflexive responses (salivation is automatic).

2) Terminology (if you are still confused by these definitions, please look in the non-Psychology jargon glossary on the AlleyDog.com homepage):

   a) Unconditioned Stimulus (US)-a stimulus that evokes an unconditioned response without any prior conditioning (no learning needed for the response to occur).

   b) Unconditioned Response (UR)-an unlearned reaction/response to an unconditioned stimulus that occurs without prior conditioning.

   c) Conditioned Stimulus (CS)-a previously neutral stimulus that has, through conditioning, acquired the capacity to evoke a conditioned response.

   d) Conditioned Response (CR)-a learned reaction to a conditioned stimulus that occurs because of prior conditioning.

   *These are reflexive behaviours. Not a result from engaging in goal directed behaviour.

e) Trial-presentation of a stimulus or pair of stimuli. Don't worry, we will get to some examples that make this all much more clear.

3) Basic Principles:

a) Acquisition-formation of a new CR tendency. This means that when an organism learns something new, it has been "acquired".

Pavlov believed in **contiguity**-temporal association between two events that occur closely together in time. The more closely in time two events occurred, the more likely they were to become associated; s time passes, association becomes less likely.

For example, when people are house training a dog — you notice that the dog went to the bathroom on the rug,. If the dog had the accident hours ago, it will not do any good to scold the dog because too much time has passed for the dog to associate your scolding with the accident. But, if you catch the dog right after the accident occurred, it is more likely to become associated with the accident.

There are several different ways conditioning can occur — order that the stimulus-response can occur:

1. **delayed conditioning (forward)-the** CS is presented before the US and it (CS) stays on until the US is presented. This is generally the best, especially when the delay is short.

   example-a bell begins to ring and continues to ring until food is presented.

2. **trace conditioning**-discrete event is presented, then the US occurs. Shorter the interval the better, but as you can tell, this approach is not very effective.

   example-a bell begins ringing and ends just before the food is presented.

3. **simultaneous conditioning**-CS and US presented together. Not very good.

   example-the bell begins to ring at the same time the food is presented. Both begin, continue, and end at the same time.

4. **backward conditioning-**US occurs before CS. example-the food is presented, then the bell rings. This is not really effective.

a) Extinction-this is a gradual weakening and eventual disappearance of the CR tendency. Extinction occurs from multiple presentations of CS without the US. Essentially, the organism continues to be presented with the conditioned stimulus but without the unconditioned stimulus the CS loses its power to evoke the CR. For example, Pavlov's dogs stopped salivating when the dispenser sound kept occurring without the meat powder following.

b) Spontaneous Recovery-sometimes there will be a reappearance of a response that had been extinguished. The recovery can occur after a period of non-exposure to the CS. It is called spontaneous because the response seems to reappear out of nowhere.

c) Stimulus Generalization-a response to a specific stimulus becomes associated to other stimuli (similar stimuli) and now occurs to those other similar stimuli. For Example-a child who gets bitten by black lab, later becomes afraid of all dogs. The original fear evoked by the Black Lab has now generalized to ALL dogs.

Another Example-little Albert (I am assuming you are familiar with Little Albert, so I will give a very general example).

d) John Watson conditioned a baby (Albert) to be afraid of a white rabbit by showing Albert the rabbit and then slamming two metal pipes together behind Albert's head (nice!). The pipes produced a very loud, sudden noise that frightened Albert and made him cry. Watson did this several times (multiple trials) until Albert was afraid of the rabbit. Previously he would pet the rabbit and play with it. After conditioning, the sight of the rabbit made Albert scream — then what Watson found was that Albert began to show similar terrified behaviours to Watson's face (just looking at Watson's face made Albert cry. What a shock!). What Watson realized was that Albert was responding to the white beard Watson had at the time. So, the fear evoked by the white, furry, rabbit, had generalized to other white, furry things, like Watson's beard.

e) Stimulus Discrimination-learning to respond to one stimulus and not another. Thus, an organisms becomes conditioned to respond to a specific stimulus and not to other stimuli.

For Example-a puppy may initially respond to lots of different people, but over time it learns to respond to only one or a few people's commands.

f) Higher Order Conditioning-a CS can be used to produce a response from another neutral stimulus (can evoke CS). There are a couple of different orders or levels. Let's take a "Pavlovian Dog-like" example to look at the different orders: In this example, light is paired with food. The food is a US since it produces a response without any prior learning. Then, when food is paired with a neutral stimulus (light) it becomes a Conditioned Stimulus (CS)-the dog begins to respond (salivate) to the light without the presentation of the food.

First order:

1) light — US (food) —> UR (salivation)

2) light — US (food) —> CR (salivation)

Second order:

3) tone — light—> CR (salivation)

4) tone — light —> CR (salivation)

Classical Conditioning in Everyday Life

One of the great things about conditioning is that we can see it all around us. Here are some examples of classical conditioning that you may see:

1. Conditioned Fear & Anxiety-many phobias that people experience are the results of conditioning.

   For Example-"fear of bridges"-fear of bridges can develop from many different sources. For example, while a child rides in a car over a dilapidated bridge, his father makes jokes about the bridge collapsing and all of them falling into the river below. The father finds this funny and so decides to do it whenever they cross the bridge. Years later, the child has grown up and now is afraid to drive over any bridge. In this case, the fear of one bridge generalized to all bridges which now evoke fear.

2. Advertising-modern advertising strategies evolved from John Watson's use of conditioning. The approach is to link an attractive US with a CS (the product being sold) so the consumer will feel positively toward the product just like they do with the US.

   US —> CS —> CR/UR

   attractive person —> car —> pleasant emotional response

3. A Clockwork Orange-No additional information necessary! If you haven't seen this movie or read the book, do it. You will find it very interesting, and a wonderful example of conditioning in action.

Operant Conditioning

Operant conditioning is the use of consequences to modify the occurrence and form of behaviour. Operant conditioning is distinguished from classical conditioning (also called respondent conditioning, or Pavlovian conditioning) in that operant conditioning deals with the modification of "voluntary behaviour" or operant behaviour. Operant behaviour "operates" on the environment and is maintained by its consequences, while classical conditioning deals with the conditioning of respondent behaviours which are elicited by antecedent conditions. Behaviours conditioned via a classical conditioning procedure are not maintained by consequences.

Reinforcement, Punishment, and Extinction

Reinforcement and punishment, the core tools of operant conditioning, are either positive (delivered following a response), or negative (withdrawn following a response). This creates a total of four basic consequences, with the addition of a fifth procedure known as extinction (i.e. no change in consequences following a response). It's important to note that organisms are not spoken of as being reinforced, punished, or extinguished; it is the response that is reinforced, punished, or extinguished. Additionally, reinforcement, punishment, and extinction are not terms whose use is restricted to the laboratory. Naturally occurring consequences can also be said to reinforce, punish, or extinguish behaviour and are not always delivered by people.

- **Reinforcement** is a consequence that causes a behaviour to occur with greater frequency.
- **Punishment** is a consequence that causes a behaviour to occur with less frequency.
- **Extinction** is the lack of any consequence following a behaviour. When a behaviour is inconsequential, producing neither favourable nor unfavourable consequences, it will occur with less frequency. When a previously reinforced behaviour is no longer reinforced with either positive or negative reinforcement, it leads to a decline in the response.

Four contexts of operant conditioning: Here the terms *"positive"* and *"negative"* are not used in their popular sense, but rather: *"positive"* refers to addition, and *"negative"* refers to subtraction. What is added or subtracted may be either reinforcement or punishment. Hence *positive punishment* is sometimes a confusing term, as it denotes the addition of punishment (such as spanking or an electric shock), a context that may seem very negative in the lay sense. The four procedures are:

1. **Positive reinforcement** occurs when a behaviour (response) is followed by a favorable stimulus (commonly seen as pleasant) that increases the frequency of that behaviour. In the Skinner box experiment, a stimulus such as food or sugar solution can be delivered when the rat engages in a target behaviour, such as pressing a lever.
2. **Negative reinforcement** occurs when a behaviour (response) is followed by the removal of an aversive

stimulus (commonly seen as unpleasant) thereby increasing that behaviour's frequency. In the Skinner box experiment, negative reinforcement can be a loud noise continuously sounding inside the rat's cage until it engages in the target behaviour, such as pressing a lever, upon which the loud noise is removed.

3. **Positive punishment** (also called "Punishment by contingent stimulation") occurs when a behaviour (response) is followed by an aversive stimulus, such as introducing a shock or loud noise, resulting in a decrease in that behaviour.
4. **Negative punishment** (also called "Punishment by contingent withdrawal") occurs when a behaviour (response) is followed by the removal of a favorable stimulus, such as taking away a child's toy following an undesired behaviour, resulting in a decrease in that behaviour.

Also:

- **Avoidance learning** is a type of learning in which a certain behaviour results in the cessation of an aversive stimulus. For example, performing the behaviour of shielding one's eyes when in the sunlight (or going indoors) will help avoid the aversive stimulation of having light in one's eyes.
- **Extinction** occurs when a behaviour (response) that had previously been reinforced is no longer effective. In the Skinner box experiment, this is the rat pushing the lever and being rewarded with a food pellet several times, and then pushing the lever again and never receiving a food pellet again. Eventually the rat would cease pushing the lever.
- **Noncontingent reinforcement** refers to delivery of reinforcing stimuli regardless of the organism's (aberrant) behaviour. The idea is that the target behaviour decreases because it is no longer necessary to receive the reinforcement. This typically entails time-based delivery of stimuli identified as maintaining aberrant behaviour, which serves to decrease the rate

of the target behaviour. As no measured behaviour is identified as being strengthened, there is controversy surrounding the use of the term noncontingent "reinforcement".

Thorndike's Law of Effect

Operant conditioning, sometimes called *instrumental conditioning* or *instrumental learning*, was first extensively studied by Edward L. Thorndike (1874-1949), who observed the behaviour of cats trying to escape from home-made puzzle boxes. When first constrained in the boxes, the cats took a long time to escape. With experience, ineffective responses occurred less frequently and successful responses occurred more frequently, enabling the cats to escape in less time over successive trials. In his Law of Effect, Thorndike theorized that successful responses, those producing *satisfying* consequences, were "stamped in" by the experience and thus occurred more frequently. Unsuccessful responses, those producing *annoying* consequences, were *stamped out* and subsequently occurred less frequently. In short, some consequences *strengthened* behaviour and some consequences *weakened* behaviour. Thorndike produced the first known learning curves through this procedure. B.F. Skinner (1904-1990) formulated a more detailed analysis of operant conditioning based on reinforcement, punishment, and extinction. Following the ideas of Ernst Mach, Skinner rejected Thorndike's mediating structures required by "satisfaction" and constructed a new conceptualization of behaviour without any such references. So while experimenting with some homemade feeding mechanisms Skinner invented the operant conditioning chamber which allowed him to measure rate of response as a key dependent variable using a cumulative record of lever presses or key pecks.

Operant Conditioning vs Fixed Action Patterns

Skinner's construct of instrumental learning is contrasted with what Nobel Prize winning biologist Konrad Lorenz termed "fixed action patterns," or reflexive, impulsive, or instinctive behaviours. These behaviours were said by Skinner and others to exist outside the parameters of operant conditioning but were considered essential to a comprehensive analysis of behaviour.

Fixed Action Patterns have their origin in the genetic makeup of the animal in question. Examples of "fixed action patterns" include ducklings that will follow any moving object if they see that object within the period of time when the behaviour will be released, or the dance that a bee performs. Characteristics of "fixed action patterns" include not needing to be learned or acquired; these behaviours are performed correctly the first time that they are performed.

Within operant conditioning, Fixed Action Patterns can be used as reinforcers for learned behaviours. Often, fixed action patterns such as predatory grabbing in dogs can be used as a reinforcer. In police and military dog training, the desire to engage in the predatory bite is often used as a reinforcement for successful completion of a search or an obedience exercise. The amount of desire that a dog might have to engage in the fixed action pattern is also known as "prey drive" although this may well be a misnomer as there is no quantification for how much a dog wants to engage in the predatory sequence.

Fixed Action Patterns can also get in the way of successful learning. Bailey and Breland note in their paper "The Mis-Behaviour of Organisms" note that raccoons cannot be taught to place an item in a jar due to the fixed action pattern that is released when they begin to place the item in the jar. When a component of a learned sequence triggers the beginning of a fixed action pattern, it is difficult and sometimes impossible to interrupt that sequence before it is completed. In this way, teaching raccoons to place items in jars, pigs to fetch (fetching triggers routing behaviours) or young ducklings to sit and stay.

Criticisms

Thorndike's law of effect specifically requires that a behaviour be followed by satisfying consequences for learning to occur. There are, however, cases in which learning can be shown to occur without good or bad effects following the behaviour. For instance, a number of experiments examining the phenomenon of latent learning showed that a rat needn't receive a satisfying reward (food, if hungry; water, if thirsty) in order to learn a maze; learning that becomes apparent immediately after the desired reward is introduced. However, views claiming such research invalidates theories of operant conditioning are molecular to a fault. If the rat has a history of "searching behaviour" being reinforced in novel environments, the behaviour will occur in new environments. This is especially plausible in a species which scavenges for food and has thus likely inherited a propensity for searching behaviour to be sensitive to reinforcement. Behaving during initial extinction trials as the organism had during reinforcement trials is not proof of latent learning, as behaviour is a function of the history of the individual organism and its genetic endowment and is never controlled by future consequences. That an organism continues to respond during unreinforced trials has been well-established when studying intermittent schedules of reinforcement.

A different experiment, in humans, showed that "punishing" the correct behaviour may actually cause it to be more frequently taken (i.e. stamp it in). Subjects are given a number of pairs of holes on a large board and required to learn which hole to poke a stylus through for each pair. If the subjects receive an electric shock for punching the correct hole, they learn which hole is correct more quickly than subjects who receive an electric shock for punching the incorrect hole. This cannot, however, be accurately described as punishment if it is increasing the probability of the behaviour.

Classical or "Pavlovian" Conditioning

Theory

Classical Conditioning is the type of learning made famous by Pavlov's experiments with dogs. The gist of the experiment is this: Pavlov presented dogs with food, and measured their salivary response (how much they drooled). Then he began ringing a bell just before presenting the food. At first, the dogs did not begin salivating until the food was presented. After a while, however, the dogs began to salivate when the sound of the bell was presented. They learned to associate the sound of the bell with the presentation of the food. As far as their immediate physiological responses were concerned, the sound of the bell became equivalent to the presentation of the food.

Classical conditioning is used by trainers for two purposes: To condition (train) autonomic responses, such as the drooling, producing adrenaline, or reducing adrenaline (calming) without using the stimuli that would naturally create such a response; and, to create an association between a stimulus that normally would not have any effect on the animal and a stimulus that would.

Stimuli that animals react to without training are called *primary* or *unconditioned stimuli* (US). They include food, pain, and other "hardwired" or "instinctive" stimuli. Animals do not have to learn to react to an electric shock, for example. Pavlov's dogs did not need to learn about food.

Stimuli that animals react to only after learning about them are called *secondary* or *conditioned stimuli* (CS). These are stimuli that have been associated with a primary stimulus. In Pavlov's experiment, the sound of the bell meant nothing to the dogs at first. After its sound was associated with the presentation of food, it became a conditioned stimulus. If a warning buzzer is associated with the shock, the animals will learn to fear it.

Secondary stimuli are things that the trainee has to learn to like or dislike. Examples include school grades and money. A slip of paper with an "A" or an "F" written on it has no meaning to a person who has never learned the meaning of the grade. Yet students work hard to gain "A's" and avoid "F's". A coin or piece of paper money has no meaning to a person who doesn't use that sort of system. Yet people have been known to work hard to gain this secondary reinforcer.

Application

Classical conditioning is very important to animal trainers, because it is difficult to supply an animal with one of the things it naturally likes (or dislikes) in time for it to be an important consequence of the behaviour. In other words, it's hard to toss a fish to a dolphin while it's in the middle of a jump or finding a piece of equipment on the ocean floor a hundred meters below. So trainers will associate something that's easier to "deliver" with something the animal wants through classical conditioning. Some trainers call this a *bridge* (because it bridges the time between when the animal performs a desired behaviour and when it gets its reward). Marine mammal trainers use a whistle. Many other trainers use a clicker, a cricket-like box with a metal tongue that makes a click-click sound when you press it.

You can classically condition a clicker by clicking it and delivering some desirable treat, many times in a row. Simply click the clicker, pause a moment, and give the dog (or other animal) the treat. After you've done this a few times, you may see the animal visibly startle, look towards the treat, or look to you. This indicates that she's starting to form the association. Some clicker trainers call this "charging up the clicker". It's also called "creating a conditioned reinforcer". The click sound becomes a signal for an upcoming reinforcement. As a shorthand, some clicker trainers will say that the click = the treat. (Read more about how to get started with clicker training here.)

Classical and Operant Conditioning

Classical Conditioning: One important type of learning, Classical Conditioning, was actually discovered accidentally by Ivan Pavlov (1849-1936). Pavlov was a Russian physiologist who discovered this phenomenon while doing research on digestion. His research was aimed at better understanding the digestive patterns in dogs. During his experiments, he would put meat powder in the mouths of dogs who had tubes inserted into various organs to measure bodily responses. What he discovered was that the dogs began to salivate before the meat powder was presented to them. Then, the dogs began to salivate as soon as the person feeding them would enter the room. He soon began to gain interest in this phenomenon and abandoned his digestion research in favour of his now famous Classical Conditioning study.

Basically, the findings support the idea that we develop responses to certain stimuli that are not naturally occurring.

When we touch a hot stove, our reflex pulls our hand back. It does this instinctually, no learning involved. It is merely a survival instinct. But why now do some people, after getting burned, pull their hands back even when the stove is not turned on? Pavlov discovered that we make associations which cause us to generalize our response to one stimuli onto a neutral stimuli it is paired with. In other words, hot burner = ouch, stove = burner, therefore, stove = ouch.

Pavlov began pairing a bell sound with the meat powder and found that even when the meat powder was not presented, the dog would eventually begin to salivate after hearing the bell. Since the meat powder naturally results in salivation, these two variables are called the unconditioned stimulus (UCS) and the unconditioned response (UCR), respectively. The bell and salivation are not naturally occurring; the dog was conditioned to respond to the bell. Therefore, the bell is considered the conditioned stimulus (CS), and the salivation to the bell, the conditioned response (CR).

Many of our behaviours today are shaped by the pairing of stimuli. Have you ever noticed that certain stimuli, such as the smell of a cologne or perfume, a certain song, a specific day of the year, results in fairly intense emotions? It's not that the smell or the song are the cause of the emotion, but rather what that smell or song has been paired with...perhaps an ex-boyfriend or ex-girlfriend, the death of a loved one, or maybe the day you met you current husband or wife. We make these associations all the time and often don't realize the power that these connections or pairings have on us. But, in fact, we have been classically conditioned.

Operant Conditioning: Another type of learning, very similar to that discussed above, is called Operant Conditioning. The term "Operant" refers to how an organism operates on the environment, and hence, operant conditioning comes from how we respond to what is presented to us in our environment. It can be thought of as learning due to the natural consequences of our actions.

Let's explain that a little further. The classic study of Operant Conditioning involved a cat who was placed in a box with only one way out; a specific area of the box had to be pressed in order for the door to open. The cat initially tries to get out of the box because freedom is reinforcing. In its attempt to escape, the area of the box is triggered and the door opens. The cat is now free. Once placed in the box again, the cat will naturally try to remember what it did to escape the previous time and will once again find the area to press. The more the cat is placed back in the box, the quicker it will press that area for its freedom. It has learned, through natural consequences, how to gain the reinforcing freedom. We learn this way every day in our lives. Imagine the last time you made a mistake; you most likely remember that mistake and do things differently when the situation comes up again. In that sense, you've learned to act differently based on the natural consequences of your previous actions. The same holds true for positive actions. If something you did results in a positive outcome, you are likely to do that same activity again.

Thorndike's Theory of Learning

1) The most basic form of learning is trial and error learning.
2) Learning is incremental not insightful.
3) Learning is not mediated by ideas.
4) All mammals learn in the same manner.
5) Law of readiness Interference with goal directed behaviour causes frustration and causing someone to do something they do not want to do is also frustrating.
   a. When someone is ready to perform some act, to do so is satisfying.
   b. When someone is ready to perform some act, not to do so is annoying.
   c. When someone is not ready to perform some act and is forced to do so, it is annoying.
6) Law of Exercise We learn by doing. We forget by not doing, although to a small extent only.
   a. Connections between a stimulus and a response are strengthened as they are used.(law of use)

b. Connections between a stimulus and a response are weakened as they are not used.(law of disuse)

7) Law of effect If the response in a connection is followed by a satisfying state of affairs, the strength of the connection is considerably increased whereas if followed by an annoying state of affairs, then the strength of the connection is marginally decreased.

8) Multiple Responses A learner would keep trying multiple responses to solve a problem before it is actually solved.

9) Set or Attitude Set or attitude is what the learner already possesses, like prior learning experiences, present state of the learner, etc., while it begins learning a new task.

10) Prepotency of Elements Different responses to the same environment would be evoked by different perceptions of the environment which act as the stimulus to the responses. Different perceptions would be subject to the prepotency of different elements for different perceivers.

11) Response from analogy New problems are solved by using solution techniques employed to solve analogous problems.

12) Associative Shifting Let stimulus S be paired with response R. Now, if stimulus Q is presented simultaneously with stimulus S repeatedly, then stimulus Q is likely to get paired with response R.

13) Belongingness If there is a natural relationship between the need state of an organism and the effect caused by a response, learning is more effective than if the relationship is unnatural.

Theory

One of Thorndike's major contributions to the study of Psychology was his work with animals. Through long, extensive research with these animals, he constructed devices called "puzzle boxes." This work on animal intelligence used equipment that became both famous and controversial. Thorndike's setup of the puzzle boxes is an example of instrumental conditioning: An animal makes some response, and if it is rewarded, the response is learned. If the response is not rewarded, it gradually disappears. The entire experiment was based on animals being placed into these contraptions, and could only escape from it by making some specific response. Such escape procedures would be pulling a sting or pushing a button.

The way his experiment worked was by placing a hungry cat into the box, then observing its behaviour as it tried to escape and obtain some food. For the most part, he noticed that the cats obtained the food only by "trial-and-error." On a successive attempt, the mere trial-and-error behaviour decreased and the cat would escape quickly. Thorndike studied several cats, and plotted the time it took for them to escape from the puzzle box on successive trials. These learning curves did not suddenly improve, but rather the amount of time the animal spent in the box gradually got to be shortened. From this, the animal did not merely realize what it had to do to escape, but the connection between the animal's situation and the response that gradually freed him was stamped in. With these observations, Thorndike suggested that certain stimuli and responses become connected or dissociated from each other according to his law of effect. He stated, "When particular stimulus-response sequences are followed by pleasure, those responses tend to be 'stamped in'; responses followed by pain tend to be 'stamped out'." The final interpretation of the law of effect was the immediate consequence of a mental connection can work back upon it to strengthen it.

This evaluation led Thorndike to conclude that animals learn, solely, by trial and error, or reward and punishment. Thorndike used the cat's behaviour in a puzzle box to describe what happens when all beings learn anything. All learning involves the formation of connections, and connections were strengthened according to the law of effect. Intelligence is the ability to form connections and humans are the most evolved animal because they form more connections then any other being. He continued his study with learning by writing his famous *Animal Intelligence*. In this he argued that we study animal behaviour, not animal consciousness, for the ultimate purpose of controlling behaviour. Today, he is known for his early animal studies and the founding principle of Instrumental Learning, "The Law of Effect".

Learning by Insight (Kohler)

Kohler's Research on the Mentality of Apes

Wolfgang Kohler, a psychologist trained at the University of Berlin, was working at a primate research facility maintained by the Prussian Academy of Sciences in the Canary Islands when the First World War broke out. Marooned there, he had at his disposal a large outdoor pen and nine chimpanzees of various ages. The pen, described by Kohler as a playground, was provided with a variety of objects including boxes, poles, and sticks, with which the primates could experiment.

Kohler constructed a variety of problems for the chimps, each of which involved obtaining food that was not directly accessible. In the simplest task, food was put on the other side of a barrier. Dogs and cats in previous experiments had faced the barrier in order to reach the food, rather than moving away from the goal to circumvent the barrier. The chimps, however, presented with an apparently analogous situation, set off immediately on the circuitous route to the food.

It is important to note that the dogs and cats that had apparently failed this test were not necessarily less intelligent than the chimps. The earlier experiments that psychologists had run on dogs and cats differed from Kohler's experiments on chimps in two important ways. First, the barriers were not familiar to the dogs and cats, and thus there was no opportunity for using latent learning, whereas the chimps were well acquainted with the rooms used in Kohler's tests. Second, whereas the food remained visible in the dog and cat experiments, in the chimp test the food was tossed out the window (after which the window was shut) and fell out of sight. Indeed, when Kohler tried the same test on a dog familiar with the room, the animal (after proving to itself that the window was shut), took the shortest of the possible indirect routes to the unseen food. The ability to select an indirect (or even novel) route to a goal is not restricted to chimps, cats, and dogs. At least some insects routinely perform similar feats. The cognitive processing underlying these abilities will become clearer when we look at navigation by chimps. For now, the point is that the chimpanzees' abilities to plan routes are not as unique as they appeared at the time.

Some of the other tests that Kohler is known for are preserved on film. In a typical sequence, a chimp jumps fruitlessly at bananas that have been hung out of reach. Usually, after a period of unsuccessful jumping, the chimp apparently becomes angry or frustrated, walks away in seeming disgust, pauses, then looks at the food in what might be a more reflective way, then at the toys in the enclosure, then back at the food, and then at the toys again. Finally the animal begins to use the toys to get at the food.

The details of the chimps' solutions to Kohler's food-gathering puzzle varied. One chimp tried to shinny up a toppling pole it had poised under the bananas; several succeeded by stacking crates underneath, but were hampered by difficulties in getting their centres of gravity right. Another chimp had good luck moving a crate under the bananas and using a pole to knock them down. The theme common to each of these attempts is that, to all appearances, the chimps were solving the problem by a kind of cognitive trial and error, as if they were experimenting in their minds before manipulating the tools. The pattern of these behaviours—failure, pause, looking at the potential tools, and then the attempt—would seem to involve insight and planning, at least on the first occasion.

Kohler's Major Contributions

During the time period, Edward Thorndike had the prevailing view of animal learning. He concluded through his studies of monkeys, dogs, and especially cats that learning is a trial-and-error process which is dependent on rewards and punishments. Kohler questioned Thorndike's conclusion that his animals learned mechanically through the selection of action of rewards and punishments (Hothersall, 1995). Kohler attempted to prove that animals arrive at a solution through insight rather than trial and error. His first experiments with dogs and cats involved food being placed on the other side of a barrier. The dogs and cats went right towards the food instead of moving away from the goal to circumvent the barrier like chimps who were presented with this situation (URL 2).

Kohler's experiments consisted of placing chimps in an enclosed area and presenting them with a reward that was out of reach, such as bananas. Kohler used four chimps in his experiments, Chica, Grande, Konsul, and Sultan. In one experiment, Kohler placed bananas outside Sultan's cage and two bamboo sticks inside his cage. Neither stick was long enough to reach the bananas so the only way to reach the bananas was to put the sticks together. Kohler demonstrated to Sultan the solution by putting his fingers into the end of one of the sticks (Hothersall, 1995). However, this did not help Sultan solve the problem. After some contemplation, Sultan put the two sticks together and created a stick long enough to reach the bananas outside his cage (URL 3).

Another study involved bananas suspended from the roof. The chimps first tried to knock them down by using a stick. Then, the chimps learned to stack boxes on top of one another to climb up to the bananas (URL 3). Kohler described three properties of insight learning. First, insight-learning is based on the animal perceiving the solution to the problem. Second, insight-leaning is not dependent on rewards. Third, once a problem has been solved, it is easier to solve a similar problem (Hothersall, 1995).

Kohler tested Gestalt theory in regards to the transposition of stimuli by training a chicken to distinguish between two shades of gray. The chicken was then rewarded for pecking at the darker gray card but was not rewarded for pecking at a lighter gray card. After numerous trials, the chicken only pecked at the darker gray card. When the chicken was exposed to a dark gray and a black card, the chicken pecked at the black card. This experiment disproves Throndike's theory that animals learn to respond to a particular stimulus with a specific response (Hothersall, 1995).

Insight Learning

The term insight refers to solving a problem through understanding the relationships of various parts of the problem. Insight often occurs suddenly, such as when a person looks at a certain problem for some time and then suddenly grasps its solution.

The psychologist Wolfgang Kohler performed important insight experiments in the early 1900's. He showed that chimpanzees sometimes use insight instead of trial-and-error responses to solve problems. When a banana was placed high out of reach, the animals discovered that they could stack boxes on top of each other to reach it. They also discovered how to put two sticks together to reach an object that was too far away to reach with one stick. The chimpanzees appeared both to see and to use the relationships involved in reaching their goals.

Theories of learning are based on facts obtained from experiments such as those on classical and instrumental conditioning. Psychologists differ in their interpretation of these facts. As a result, there are a number of learning theories. These theories can be divided into three groups.

One group of psychologists emphasizes stimulus-response relationships and has performed experiments with classical and instrumental conditioning. They say all learning is the forming of habits. When we learn, we connect a stimulus and a response that did not exist before, thus forming a habit. Habits can range from the simplest ones to complex ones that are involved in learning skills. These psychologists believe that when we meet a new problem, we use appropriate responses learned from past experience to solve it. If this procedure does not lead to the solution, we use a trial-and-error approach. We use one response after another until we solve the problem. The stimulus-response approach has been used to explain and modify bad habits. For example, when a person is irrationally afraid of dogs, methods called behaviour modification can be used to replace the fear response to a dog with a more relaxed response.

A second group of psychologists stresses cognition (the act of knowing) above the importance of habit. These experts feel that experiments with classical and instrumental conditioning are too limited to explain such complex learning as understanding concepts and ideas. This approach emphasizes the importance of the learner's discovering and perceiving new relationships and achieving insight and understanding.

A third group of psychologists has developed humanistic theories. According to these theories, much human learning results from the need to express creativity. Almost any activity, including athletics, business dealings, and homemaking, can serve as a creative outlet. The psychologists in this group believe that each person must become involved in challenging activities—and must do reasonably well at them—to have a satisfying life. The individual gains a sense of control, growth, and knowledge from such activities. For learning to occur, people must feel free to make their own decisions. They also must feel worthy, relatively free from anxiety, self-respecting, and respected by others. Under these conditions, their own inner drives will lead them to learn. Some kinds of group therapy try to provide an accepting, supporting environment. Such an environment is intended to increase people's awareness of their own thoughts and of the world around them.

Learning involves changes in the nervous system. Scientists are trying to discover the processes that take place in the brain to produce learning. Such research may lead to a physiological theory of learning.

Transfer of Training

Psychologists and educators recognize that new learning can profit from old learning because learning one thing helps in learning something else. This process is called transfer of training. Transfer of training can be either positive or negative. Suppose a person learns two tasks. After learning Task 1, the person might find Task 2 easier or harder. If Task 2 is easier, then the old learning has been a help and positive transfer of training has occurred. If Task 2 is harder, the old learning is a hindrance and negative transfer has occurred.

Whether transfer is positive or negative depends on the relationship between the two tasks. Positive transfer occurs when the two tasks have similar stimuli and both stimuli elicit the same response. For example, if we know the German word gross, it is easier to learn the French word gros because both words mean large. In this case, similar stimuli (gross and gros) elicit the same response (large).

Negative transfer occurs when the two tasks have similar stimuli, which elicit different responses. After you learn the German word Gras (grass), it is harder to learn the French word gras (fat). The words are spelled the same way, but they have different meanings. In this case, similar stimuli (Gras and gras) elicit different responses.

Psychologists believe new learning can profit from old learning because of three factors: (1) positive transfer of training, (2) general principles that we learn in one task and apply to another task, and (3) good study habits that we learn in one task which help us learn another task.

Transfer of Learning

Transfer (of learning) research can be loosely framed as the study of the dependency of human conduct on prior experience. The notion was originally introduced as *transfer of practice* by Edward Thorndike and Robert S. Woodworth (1901). They explored how individuals would transfer learning in one context to another context that shared similar characteristics. Their theory implied that transfer of learning depends on the proportion to which the learning task and the transfer task are identical, also known as 'identical elements'. Transfer research has since attracted much attention in numerous domains, producing a wealth of empirical findings and theoretical interpretations. However, there remains considerable controversy about how transfer of learning should be conceptualized and explained, what its relation is to learning, or whether it exists at all (e.g., Detterman, 1993; Helfenstein, 2005).

Transfer of learning should not be confused with knowledge transfer, as the former concerns intra-individual, constructivist perspective, and the latter, an inter-individual or inter-organizational perspective.

Most discussions of transfer to date can be developed from a common operational definition, describing it as the process and the effective extent to which past experiences (also referred to as transfer source) affect learning and performance in a present novel situation (transfer target) (Ellis, 1965; Woodworth, 1938). This, however, is usually also where the general consensus between various research approaches ends.

Indeed, there is a wide variety of viewpoints taken on transfer; and therefore research should be reviewed from many different perspectives. These perspectives relate to:

- a taxonomical approach to transfer research that usually intends to categorize transfer into different types;
- an application domain-driven approach by focusing on developments and contributions of different disciplines that have traditionally been interested in transfer;
- the examinination of the psychological scope of transfer models with respect to the psychological functions or faculties that are being regarded; and
- a concept-driven evaluation, which reveals underlying relationships and differences between theoretical and empirical traditions.

Learning by Imitation

Learning by Imitation: Let us now turn to the other side of the question. Let us consider the case in which the power of performing an action is acquired in and by the process of imitation itself. Here there is a general rule which is obvious when once it is pointed out. It is part of the still more general rule that "to him that hath shall be given." Our power of imitating the activity of another is strictly proportioned to our preexisting power of performing the same general kind of action independently.

For instance, one who is devoid of musical faculty has practically no power of imitating the violin playing of Joachim. Imitation may develop and improve a power which already exists, but it cannot create it. Consider the child beginning for the first time to write in a copybook. He learns by imitation;

but it is only because he has already some rudimentary ability to make such simple figures as pothooks that the imitative process can get a start. At the outset, his pothooks are very unlike the model set before him. Gradually he improves; increased power of independent production gives step by step increased power ot imitation, until he approaches too closely the limits of his capacity in this direction to make any further progress of an appreciable kind.

But this is an incomplete account of the matter. The power of learning by imitation is part of the general power of learning by experience; it involves mental plasticity. An animal which starts life with congenital tendencies and aptitudes of a fixed and stereotyped kind, so that they admit of but little modification in the course of individual development, has correspondingly little power of learning by imitation. Among animals, monkeys have the greatest plasticity and the greatest aptitude for imitation.

They are incessantly active in all kinds of ways, and they are in a very high degree capable of learning by experience. T' us, when admitted to the company of human beings, they will spontaneously learn the use of knives, forks, cups, plates, etc. In general, the more intelligent monkeys have a wider and more varied sphere of activity than other animals. They are incessantly trying to do things, experimenting in all sorts of ways, and learning rapidly by the success or failure of their attempts. The wide range of their activity involves a wide range of interest. They attend to all kinds of things without any directly practical aim; and the imitative impulse is, as we have seen, a special development of this form of attention. The readiest way of bringing before their consciousness vividly and distinctly an action which interests them, is to reenact it themselves.

Of course at higher levels of mental development the imitative impulse is far less conspicuous because impulsive activity in general is checked and overruled by activity organised in a unified system.* Civilised men imitate not so much because of immediate interest in the action imitated as with a view to the attainment of desirable results.

Levels of Learning-Gagne

Gagne's Instructional Design Theory

Introduction to Gagne: Gagne's work has been particularly influential in training and the design of instructional materials. In fact, the idea that instruction can be systematically designed can be attributed to Gagne and a handful of others. It's interesting to speculate how his early work in Air Force training may have shaped his theory. I wonder if it might have evolved differently had he been working with college students, or 3rd graders?

Be sure you understand the difference between theories of learning and theories of instruction. The Driscoll chapter does a pretty good job of explaining this.

Gagne's instructional theory has three major elements. First, it is based on a *taxonomy, or classification, of learning outcomes*. Second, it proposes particular *internal and external conditions* necessary for achieving these learning outcomes. And third, it offers nine *events of instruction*, which serve as a template for developing and delivering a unit of instruction.

Gagne's Taxonomy of Learning Outcomes

The notion of different "levels" of learning or knowing something is a very useful one in education. You have probably been in or observed a class where the teacher said she or he wanted to help student achieve high-level skills such as being able to analyze problems, evaluate cases, etc.; but when you looked at the test items for the class, they mostly had to do with memorizing terms and definitions. This is a "learning-levels" problem.

For example, what does it mean to ask if someone "knows" a concept such as "analysis of variance," (ANOVA) the statistical procedure that most of us have encountered—or will? Do we want to know if they can

- state or write the formula for ANOVA?
- explain what the formula means?
- use the formula correctly when told to do so?

- know *when* to use it, without being told?
- know how to interpret the results? etc., etc.

Gagne and others thought it was important for teachers and instructional designers to think carefully about the nature of the skill or task they wanted to teach, then to make sure that the learner had the necessary prerequisites to acquire that skill. Gagne also stressed that practice and assessment should match the target skill. In other words, if we want someone to know when to use an ANOVA, and be able to use it to answer real questions, then it is of little use to test them on their ability to write the formula.

Of the four categories of learning outcomes Gagne proposes, the one that seems to have gotten the most attention is *intellectual skills.* It is important to understand that the five sub-categories of intellectual skills are believed to be hierarchical. That is, for a given skill at, say, the level of "defined concepts," there should be underlying discriminations and concrete concepts that must first be mastered.

According to Gagne's theory, the way to determine the prerequisites for a given learning objective is to conduct a *learning hierarchy.* A learning hierarchy (sometimes called a task analysis) is constructed by working backwards from the final learning objective. Suppose, for example, that the desired learning outcome is to be able to be able to balance one's checkbook upon receiving the monthly bank statement. We would ask ourselves, what are the component skills of balancing a checkbook?

They might include things such as, identifying the relevant information on the bank statement, accurately entering deductions and deposits in the check register, and knowing to add back to one's ending balance any outstanding checks in order to reconcile the checkbook balance with that indicated on the bank statement. Assuming we decided that these were, in fact, the three component skills, we would then need to analyze each of these into more basic component skills. How many levels "deep" would we need to go in such a hierarchy? One answer to that question would be, until we reach the level of skills that we know the target learners already possess.

Conditions of Learning (R. Gagne)

Overview: This theory stipulates that there are several different types or **levels** of learning. The significance of these classifications is that each different type requires different types of instruction. Gagne identifies five major categories of learning: verbal information, intellectual skills, cognitive strategies, motor skills and attitudes. Different internal and external conditions are necessary for each type of learning. For example, for cognitive strategies to be learned, there must be a chance to practice developing new solutions to problems; to learn attitudes, the learner must be exposed to a credible role model or persuasive arguments. Gagne suggests that learning tasks for intellectual skills can be organized in a hierarchy according to complexity: stimulus recognition, response generation, procedure following, use of terminology, discriminations, concept formation, rule application, and problem solving. The primary significance of the hierarchy is to identify prerequisites that should be completed to facilitate learning at each level. Prerequisites are identified by doing a task analysis of a learning/training task. Learning hierarchies provide a basis for the sequencing of instruction.

In addition, the theory outlines nine instructional events and corresponding cognitive processes:

(1) gaining attention (reception)
(2) informing learners of the objective (expectancy)
(3) stimulating recall of prior learning (retrieval)
(4) presenting the stimulus (selective perception)
(5) providing learning guidance (semantic encoding)
(6) eliciting performance (responding)
(7) providing feedback (reinforcement)
(8) assessing performance (retrieval)
(9) enhancing retention and transfer (generalization).

These events should satisfy or provide the necessary conditions for learning and serve as the basis for designing instruction and selecting appropriate media (Gagne, Briggs & Wager, 1992).

Scope/Application: While Gagne's theoretical framework covers all aspects of learning, the focus of the theory is on intellectual skills. The theory has been applied to the design of instruction in all domains (Gagner & Driscoll, 1988). In its original formulation (Gagne, 1 962), special attention was given to military training settings. Gagne (1987) addresses the role of instructional technology in learning.

Remembering and Forgetting—Curve of Forgetting

Forgetting: When Memory Fails

From forgetting where you left your keys to forgetting to return a phone call, memory failures are an almost daily occurrence. Forgetting is so common that we typically rely on numerous methods to help us remember important information, such as jotting down notes in a daily planner or scheduling important events in your Blackberry calendar. As you are frantically searching for your missing car keys, it may seem that the information about where you left them is permanently gone from your memory. However, forgetting is generally not about actually losing or erasing this information from your long-term memory. Forgetting typically involves a failure in memory retrieval. While the information is somewhere in your long-term memory, you are not able to actually retrieve and remember it.

The Ebbinghaus Forgetting Curve

Psychologist Hermann Ebbinghaus was one of the first to scientifically study forgetting. In experiments where is used himself as the subject, Ebbinghaus tested his memory using three-letter nonsense syllables. Using previously known words would have made use of previously existing knowledge and association in his memory. In order to test his memory for new information, Ebbinghaus tested his memory for periods of time ranging from 20 minutes to 31 days. He then published his findings in 1885 in *Memory: A Contribution to Experimental Psychology*. His results, plotted in what is known as the Ebbinghaus forgetting curve, revealed a relationship between forgetting and time. Initially, information is often lost very quickly after it is learned. Factors such as how the information was learned and how frequently it was rehearsed play a role in how quickly these memories are lost. The forgetting curve also showed that forgetting does not continue to decline until all of the information is lost. At a certain point, the amount of forgetting levels off. What exactly does this mean? It indicates that information stored in long-term memory is surprisingly stable.

Measures of Forgetting and Retention

Researchers measure forgetting and retention in three different ways: recall, recognition, and relearning.

Recall

Recall is remembering without any external cues. For example, essay questions test recall of knowledge because nothing on a blank sheet of paper will jog the memory.

Recognition

Recognition is identifying learned information using external cues. For example, true or false questions and multiple-choice questions test recognition because the previously learned information is there on the page, along with other options. In general, recognition is easier than recall.

Relearning

When using the **relearning** method to measure retention, a researcher might ask a subject to memorize a long grocery list. She might measure how long he has to practice before he remembers every item. Suppose it takes him ten minutes. On another day, she gives him the same list again and measures how much time he takes to relearn the list. Suppose he now learns it in five minutes. He has saved five minutes of learning time, or 50 percent of the original time it took him to learn it. His savings score of 50 percent indicates that he retained 50 percent of the information he learned the first time.

Causes of Forgetting

Everyone forgets things. There are six main reasons for forgetting: ineffective encoding, decay, interference, retrieval failure, motivated forgetting, and physical injury or trauma.

Ineffective Encoding

The way information is **encoded** affects the ability to remember it. Processing information at a deeper level makes it harder to forget. If a student thinks about the meaning of the concepts in her textbook rather than just reading them, she'll remember them better when the final exam comes around. If the information is not encoded properly—such as if the student simply skims over the textbook while paying more attention to the TV—it is more likely to be forgotten.

Decay

According to **decay theory**, memory fades with time. Decay explains the loss of memories from sensory and short-term memory. However, loss of long-term memories does not seem to depend on how much time has gone by since the information was learned. People might easily remember their first day in junior high school but completely forget what they learned in class last Tuesday.

Interference

Interference theory has a better account of why people lose long-term memories. According to this theory, people forget information because of interference from other learned information. There are two types of interference: retroactive and proactive.

- **Retroactive interference** happens when newly learned information makes people forget old information.
- **Proactive interference** happens when old information makes people forget newly learned information.

Retrieval Failure

Forgetting may also result from failure to **retrieve** information in memory, such as if the wrong sort of **retrieval cue** is used. For example, Dan may not be able to remember the name of his fifth-grade teacher. However, the teacher's name might suddenly pop into Dan's head if he visits his old grade school and sees his fifth-grade classroom. The classroom would then be acting as a context cue for retrieving the memory of his teacher's name.

Motivated Forgetting

Psychologist **Sigmund Freud** proposed that people forget because they push unpleasant or intolerable thoughts and feelings deep into their unconscious. He called this phenomenon **repression**. The idea that people forget things they don't want to remember is also called **motivated forgetting** or psychogenic amnesia.

Physical Injury or Trauma

Anterograde amnesia is the inability to remember events that occur after an injury or traumatic event. **Retrograde amnesia** is the inability to remember events that occurred before an injury or traumatic event.

The Curve of Forgetting

In the late 1800s, a German scientist named Ebbinghaus experimented with memory by creating lists of nonsense syllables (huf jeik mek meun pon...) and measuring how long it took to forget and then relearn them. In 1885, he published *Memory: A Contribution to Experimental Psychology* which became part of a new area of study.

He discovered some regularities that allowed him to create some "laws" of memory. He was to draw a learning curve-something that had not been done before. He called one phenomenon he observed "the spacing effect." His theory was that you could significantly improve learning by "correctly" spacing the study sessions. Should you cram for the exam, pull an all-nighter, or study a little bit every day for a week before the test?

This lesson in psych history came to me by way of an article in Wired about Piotr Wozniak. Though it's an article on memory (in an issue about being smarter), what it get me thinking about more than remembering is forgetting.

We have all read or heard that all those things we have experienced and learned are in there somewhere, and the problem is getting access to that little piece of our brain. So, maybe what we need to figure out as learners (students & teachers) is not how to learn but how to not forget.

Piotr Wozniak is a Polish biologist and computer scientist who has been working on techniques to improve memory and learning following the path first opened by Ebbinghaus. He is the inventor of a technique now contained in a software program called SuperMemo.

SuperMemo (as in super *memo*ry not memorandums) has many people using it worldwide, particularly for learning languages. It's popular enough to have the dubious honour of being pirated on bulletin boards in China and being illegally cloned with titles like *Sugar*Memo.

SuperMemo is based on the idea that there is an ideal moment to reinforce or practice what you have previously learned. If you do that next session too soon, you're wasting the effort. Wait too long and you have forgotten enough that it relearning again.

In Wozniak-speak, Supermemo "predicts the future state of a person's memory and schedules information reviews at the optimal time."

So what is the magic moment? It's at that moment when you are just about to forget. Of course, the problem is finding that moment which varies depending on the type of information and the person learning it.

The *Wired* article uses this analogy: "Imagine a pile of thousands of flash cards. Somewhere in this pile are the ones you should be practicing right now. Which are they?"

The graph shown here isn't Ebbinghaus' learning curve, but a **curve of forgetting**. Apparently, it's not new to cognitive psychology. What is new is applying it in some practical way to improving learning.

Supermemo.net is an online version that you can sign up for access in both a pay and free version.

What can we discover from SuperMemo? Let's say we are learning new vocabulary. If we know that our ability to recall a word declines over time according to a predictable forgetting curve, we use the program to remind us to review.

When you first learn that new word, your chance of recalling drops quickly, but if you are reminded at the right times the rate of forgetting levels out. If you (or a program) can track this new decline, you can wait longer next time to review (rehearse? quiz? test?) again.

Wozniak is still at it. He started 9 years ago to keep a detailed record of his sleep. Now he's trying to correlate that data with his daily performance on study repetitions because psychologists believe there's a correlation between sleep and memory, buthaven't been able to discover a mathematical law for it.

Unfortunately, most learners don't have Supermemo around all day to keep reminding them to study. And if we did have those reminders, would we be motivated to take heed of them?

The Wired article first suggests:

"The problem of forgetting might not torment us so much if we could only convince ourselves that remembering isn't important. Perhaps the things we learn words, dates, formulas, historical and biographical details don't really matter. Facts can be looked up. That's what the Internet is for. When it comes to learning, what really matters is how things fit together. We master the stories, the schemas, the frameworks, the paradigms; we rehearse the lingo; we swim in the episteme."

That's comforting to aging brains like mine. Too bad it's false.

"The people who criticize memorization" how happy would they be to spell out every letter of every word they read?" asks Robert Bjork, chair of UCLA's psychology department and one of the most eminent memory researchers. After all, Bjork notes, children learn to read whole words through intense practice, and every time we enter a new field we become children again. "You can't escape memorization," he says. "There is an initial process of learning the names of things. That's

a stage we all go through. It's all the more important to go through it rapidly."

I think we all overdo the brain as computer analogy. The brain is far more amazing than anything we will ever build. Still, we do need to load that data into memory to make the associations and do the processing down the line.

Memory Loss: Forgetting

Forgetting is the loss or failure of memory. Hermann Ebbinghaus studied the relationship between ease of relearning (called savings) and the time between learning and relearning, which he expressed as a forgetting curve. He found that most forgetting occurs during the first nine hours after learning.

Practice, both **massed** and **distributed** over time, also affects relearning forgotten material. Ebbinghaus also found that the more an individual rehearses a list of syllables, the better the syllables are recalled. (And as would be expected, given the primacy and recency effects, syllables near the beginning or end of a list are recalled best.) When graphed, the effect of practice results in a U-shaped curve.

Measures of retention. Memories may be retrieved in three ways.

- **recall**: remembering of previously learned information
    - o **free recall**: recall of items in any order
    - o **serial recall**: recall of items in the order in which they were learned
    - o **paired associate recall**: recall of a second item based on a cue supplied by a first item
- **recognition**: identification of previously learned information (as, for example from a number of answer choices in a multiple-choice test)
- **reconstruction**: rebuilding of a scenario from certain remembered details

Reasons for Forgetting

- **Decay** is loss of information from memory as a consequence of die passage of time and lack of use. It has been suggested that memory is stored in **memory traces**, which disappear when not used for a long time.

- **Interference** is the confusion of one piece of information with another or the suppression of one in favour of another that was processed about the same time (as might happen, for example, if a student takes a Spanish lesson one period and a French lesson the next).
  - o **Proactive interference** occurs if previously learned material interferes with learning of new material.
  - o **Retroactive interference** occurs if learning of new material interferes with the ability to recall previously learned material.
- **Amnesia** is the inability to remember events from the past because of a psychological trauma (**psychogenic amnesia**) or a physiological trauma (**organic amnesia**), such as brain damage resulting from a blow to the head. The memory loss is usually limited to a specific period.
  - o **Retrograde amnesia** is the inability to remember happenings that preceded the traumatic event producing the amnesia.
  - o **Anterograde amnesia** is the inability to remember happenings that occur after a traumatic event.
- People sometimes forget things because they find them too unpleasant to think about. Such an occurrence is called **motivated forgetting.** Sigmund Freud attributed many memory failures, particularly involving painful childhood experiences, to **repression** (the process of keeping disturbing thoughts or feelings relegated to the unconscious). The repressed material can sometimes be recalled through free association or hypnosis. The recovery of supposedly repressed memories, such as those of childhood sexual abuse, is controversial. Some psychologists, such as Elizabeth Loftus, have called some of the recovered

information **false memories** and suggested that sometimes such information has been implanted by the client's therapist.

Eyewitness testimony. Eyewitness testimony is the courtroom recall of a real-life situation. Studies have shown that eyewitnesses sometimes recall events incorrectly or identify the wrong people.

In addition, memories may be embellished after the fact, particularly if a person has a stake in the outcome, but although the memories seemingly improve with time, they may be less rather than more accurate. The reliability of such embellished memories is controversial as is the use of hypnosis to improve memory retrieval.

Unit-VI

Intelligence and Creativity

Individual Differences

The science of psychology studies people at three levels of focus captured by the well known quote: "Every man is in certain respects (a) like all other men, (b) like some other men, (c) like no other man" (Murray, H.A. & C. Kluckhohn, 1953).

Individual differences psychology focuses on this second level of study. It is also sometimes called Differential Psychology because researchers in this area study the ways in which individual people differ in their behaviour. This is distinguished from other aspects of psychology in that although psychology is ostensibly a study of individuals, modern psychologists often study groups or biological underpinnings of cognition.

For example, in evaluating the effectiveness of a new therapy, the mean performance of the therapy in one group might be compared to the mean effectiveness of a placebo (or a well-known therapy) in a second, control group.

In this context, differences between individuals in their reaction to the experimental and control manipulations are actually treated as errors rather than as interesting phenomena to study.

This is because psychological research depends upon statistical controls that are only defined upon groups of people. Individual difference psychologists usually express their interest in individuals while studying groups by seeking dimensions shared by all individuals but upon which individuals differ.

Nature of Intelligence

Intelligence is the *manipulation of motor mechanisms* to derive happiness for the organism – inclusive of surviving – and entails the gathering of information external to the organism so by nonverbal communication and wise *motor manipulation*, it can maximize happiness. And, at root, all living organisms are nothing more than a physical organization of their genotype: the initial genetic blueprint of an organism. Ultimately, at its root, the genotype is actually nothing more than immaterial energy configuring atoms and molecules into genetic code. As it is immaterial – as a thought or idea is immaterial – the genotype is more like a "thought" or "idea" interacting with the other "thoughts" and "ideas" and set to interact in harmony with its environment – also a "thought." Interaction is a *"thought being thought-out."* This idea is not new nor original. Aristotle theorized that God was pure Thought and prior to the Greeks, the Judeo-Christian idea of the Logos, and Egyptian idea of their God, Amun.

The physical is not the blueprint – the immaterial electromagnetic is. The immaterial is idea-like – a living *thought*. As thinking is mediated by plus and minus ions ($NaCl^-$, KCl^-, NA^+, K^+, Cl^-) moving in and out of the nerve fibres of our brain and nervous system, *thought* and *thinking* is the sophisticated summation of the flows and interplay of positive and negative energies. Both the medium for thinking (i.e. the brain) and the ability of thinking itself exist in "seed-like" form in the genotype and is "species-specific."

The nature of the genotype is that it is a *hand-glove model* of its environment both in the sense that all features of a given animal's environment are modelled in the genotype's blueprint and in that the genotype creates the animal's body and behaviour to fit *hand-glove* into its unique environment. In essence, in tiny cells, genotypes taken as a whole – at some snapshot of geological time – serve as a perfect multimedia picture-record written, imprinted in genetic code, of the heavens, the skies, the waters, and the living earth. Paul Davies, writing of the ability of birds to use stars in their astro-navigation, comments that, "The necessary astro-navigational information is built in

DNA... given a sufficient understanding of the nature of DNA, one could 'decode' this information and reconstruct a map of the stars." DNA is built on an immaterial blueprint.

In the case of you and I, we are, in essence, just the immaterial blueprint of the one-celled genotype that became us: eyes, brain, charming smile, wit, and great brilliance included. Language ability is nothing more than the ability of the genotype to associate random sounds with contemporary objects of evolution (i.e. today's world is different from the first human's world). Reading and writing is nothing less than the ability of the genome to devise and associate random signs (otherwise known as written alphabets, words, and languages) with contemporary objects of evolution such as the words "ice cream" and the "Internet." Rats evolve right along with us finding great comfort in living structures and types of food the prehistoric world had no imagination would ever exist. Insects have also kept pace with human evolution. Even viruses: computer viruses.

We are living witnesses of co-evolution. We can observe the ability of organisms worldwide to harmoniously co-evolve ever upwards: e.g. in the microscopic-level arm's race, viral innovations against medicines force humans to develop better medicines. Harmonious tit for tat co-evolution finds origins in the organizational marvel of the immaterial dimension. One unfortunate effect of imbalance is that it creates new "harmonious" balances and the imbalances the human has produced have eliminated many life forms from the environment that man is destroying in 200 years that took 2 million years to create.

Nevertheless, for living creatures, harmony and balance with nature are written and achieved in genotypes and together, genotypes make the whole living picture of life on earth – each specie of genotype one piece of the puzzle fitting perfectly with the rest. With the right equipment, the genotype could play an organism's life like a video in a VCR. Through life – via the interaction of living things – Nature manifests on yet another level, the balance and harmony found throughout the universe. Balance is found, for instance, in every animal having a strength of defense against others, but a weakness making it available as fodder and the strong have the greatest liklihood of surviving, but death takes an old life away to make way for new.

While from the perspective of the individual, intelligence serves the purpose of striving for, realizing, and maintaining individual happiness, taken as a whole intelligence serves the greater purpose of bringing the whole of the living world and nature into harmonious oneness. Let us remember several things: living things have not the foggiest idea of the technologies that make their organs and forms and make them interact harmoniously within the organism and with the whole environment from starlight to raindrops.

Differences in Intelligence

In this module, we will consider the extremes of intelligence— from the very bright to the very dull. We will also look at a few of the many studies that have been done with IQ scores, correlating many things from sense of humour (Brumbaugh, 1939) to racial background. A few of these correlation studies and their results will be described in this module. As you read the text, try to answer the following questions.

- When is a child considered gifted? Retarded?
- What are the degrees of mental retardation?
- What were Terman's findings in his study of gifted children?
- How does intelligence correlate with sex? Race? Socioeconomic level?

Distribution of Intelligence

People who score above 130 on intelligence tests are usually considered gifted. An important study of gifted children was undertaken by who devised the Stanford-Binet test. In the course of developing that test, Terman and his associates tested many thousands of children, and then did further research on those who had lO's of 140 or more. This group of more than 1500 children was in the top 1% of the population. Terman followed most of these children from 1921 until his death in

1956. Some of his associates are still continuing this detailed longitudinal study. The study revealed an important fact related to the home environments of the children. Approximately one-third were children of professional people and about half were children of persons in business occupations. Only seven percent came from "working classes." These percentages do not agree at ail with the distribution of social class membership in the general population. They indicate that relatively more gifted children come from the higher socioeconómic classes, although they do not tell us why.

Another discovery in Terman's study was that gifted children are more successful in later life. Twenty-five years after the study began, about 700 of the original group were still in contact with Terman. Of these, 150 were considered very successful. This distinction was based on such criteria as being listed in Who's Who or having received recognition for outstanding intellectual or professional achievement. Most of the others were much more successful than people of average intelligence. On the other hand, some persons in the gifted group had committed crimes, dropped out of school early, or been unsuccessful at a number of jobs. Those least successful were more poorly adjusted emotionally and less motivated than the others. On the whole, though, the most striking fact revealed in the study was that gifted children made generally outstanding contributions to society in the form of intellectual achievements.

In their early years, Terman's gifted children were above average in height, weight, and physical development, and they were also better adjusted. It had ben generally believed that very gifted children were likely to be maladjusted and socially backward. Terman's study definitely disproved this notion.

The gifted child is liable to encounter serious difficulties in school. He may be bored by children of his own age and his knowledge may even exceed that of his teacher. Teachers may consider him rude or a show-off. He may become a real problem simply because he is bored and loses interest in a class designed for "average" children. Some schools today are facing this problem by planning appropriate programs for gifted children.

Theory of Intelligences: Single, Two Factor and Multifactor Theories

The **theory of multiple intelligences** was proposed by Howard Gardner in 1983, to more accurately define the concept of intelligence and address whether methods which claim to measure intelligence (or aspects thereof) are truly scientific.

Gardner's theory argues that intelligence, particularly as it is traditionally defined, does not sufficiently encompass the wide variety of abilities humans display. In his conception, a child who masters multiplication easily is not necessarily more intelligent *overall* than a child who struggles to do so. The second child may be stronger in another *kind* of intelligence, and therefore may best learn the given material through a different approach, may excel in a field outside of mathematics, or may even be looking through the multiplication learning process at a fundamentally deeper level that hides a potentially higher mathematical intelligence than in the one who memorizes the concept easily.

Development of the Theory

"Howard Gardner, multiple intelligences and education" by given field (child prodigies, autistic savants);

- Neurological evidence for areas of the brain that are specialized for particular capacities (often including studies of people who have suffered brain damage affecting a specific capacity);
- The evolutionary relevance of the various capacities;
- Psychometric studies; and
- Susceptibility to encoding in a symbol system or notation (e.g. written language, musical notation, choreography).
- An identifiable core operation or set of operations.
- A distinctive development history, along with a definable set of 'end-state' performances.

Gardner originally identified seven core intelligences: linguistic, logical-mathematical, spatial, bodily-kinesthetic, musical, interpersonal and intrapersonal. In 1997 at the symposium "MIND 97" (Multiple Intelligences New Directions) he added an eighth, the "Naturalist" Intelligence. Investigation continues on whether there are Existentialist (existential) and Spiritualist (spiritual) Intelligences.

The theory has been widely criticized in the psychology and educational theory communities. The most common criticisms argue that Gardner's theory is based on his own intuition rather than empirical data and that the intelligences are just other names for talents or personality types. Despite these criticisms, the theory has enjoyed a great deal of popularity amongst educators over the past twenty years. There are several schools which espouse MI as a pedagogy, and many individual teachers who incorporate some or all of the theory into their methodology. Many books and educational materials exist which explain the theory and how it may be applied to the classroom.

Guilford's 'Structure of Intellect'

Structure of Intellect's System (SOI) is the basis of our academic/educational assessment.

Based on J. P. Guilford's theory of multiple intelligence and developed by Mary Meeker for use in schools, SOI tests a range of abilities (intelligences) which are needed for success with academic studies as well as in the work place. Mary Meeker found that intelligence is not "fixed", it can be developed. Upon diagnosing strengths and weaknesses, SOI's follow-up program builds potential abilities to enable success in school and in life. This program has wide-ranging applications in reading readiness, academic assessment and remediation, and career counselling.

Structure of Intellect (SOI) is a theory of human intelligence that was developed from Dr. J.P. Guilford's work at the University of Southern California. A psychologist in the U.S. Air Force in mid 1900s, Guilford created his assessment tool to help the Air Force find pilots who would succeed in the field. Despite other types of screening tests such as those for IQ and aptitude, 30% of the trainees did not make it through their vocational training. Upon putting his theories to practice, the attrition rate dropped dramatically. Guildford's assessment was adapted from his theory of multiple intelligence, which proposed 150 different abilities, extrapolated from his three dimensional model.

Dr. Mary Meeker, at the time a student of Guilford's and a psychologist, saw the potential of Guilford's work for use in the educational field, and modified his model to become an assessment and remediation tool for students in the educational system. Her adapted version (SOI) also showed potential in career counselling and the development of foundational cognitive skills needed in the workplace.

The success of this model has proved itself. SOI is currently being used in schools and learning clinics in North America to diagnose and remediate learning disabilities in students, as well as for enrichment of gifted students. The program is also implemented in employment training programs and in business and industry.

Structure of Intellect's philosophy is that intelligence is not "fixed", as has been generally supposed. Intellectual abilities can be taught. With the advent of studies in the plasticity of the brain, researchers have brought this new awareness into the fields of neuroscience and education. IQ tests have traditionally been slanted towards measuring a narrow range of abilities. Structure of Intellect's test measures a wide range of abilities needed for academic success.

Although the ability to pinpoint problem areas is highly valuable, the results would not be as effective without a corresponding system in place to remediate these areas. Structure of Intellect's diagnostic test leads directly to remediation by developing potential learning abilities.

Gardner's Multiple Intelligence Theory

The categories of intelligence proposed by Gardner are:

Bodily-kinesthetic

This area has to do with bodily movement. In theory, people who have Bodily-kinesthetic intelligence should learn better by involving muscular movement, i.e. getting up and moving around into the learning experience, and are generally good at physical activities such as sports or dance. They may enjoy acting or performing, and in general they are good at building and making things. They often learn best by doing something physically, rather than reading or hearing about it. Those with strong bodily-kinesthetic intelligence seem to use what might be termed muscle memory-they remember things through their body such as verbal memory or images.

Careers that suit those with this intelligence include athletes, dancers, actors, surgeons, doctors, builders, and soldiers. Although these careers can be duplicated through virtual simulation they will not produce the actual physical learning that is needed in this intelligence.

Interpersonal

This area has to do with interaction with others. In theory, people who have a high interpersonal intelligence tend to be extroverts, characterized by their sensitivity to others' moods, feelings, temperaments and motivations, and their ability to cooperate in order to work as part of a group. They communicate effectively and empathize easily with others, and may be either leaders or followers. They typically learn best by working with others and often enjoy discussion and debate.

Careers that suit those with this intelligence include sales, politicians, managers, teachers, and social workers.

Verbal-linguistic

This area has to do with words, spoken or written. People with high verbal-linguistic intelligence display a facility with words and languages. They are typically good at reading, writing, telling stories and memorizing words along with dates. They tend to learn best by reading, taking notes, listening to lectures, and discussion and debate. They are also frequently skilled at explaining, teaching and oration or persuasive speaking. Those with verbal-linguistic intelligence learn foreign languages very easily as they have high verbal memory and recall, and an ability to understand and manipulate syntax and structure.

This intelligence is highest in writers, lawyers, philosophers, journalists, politicians, poets, and teachers.

Logical-mathematical

This area has to do with logic, abstractions, reasoning, and numbers. While it is often assumed that those with this intelligence naturally excel in mathematics, chess, computer programming and other logical or numerical activities, a more accurate definition places emphasis on traditional mathematical ability and more reasoning capabilities, abstract patterns of recognition, scientific thinking and investigation, and the ability to perform complex calculations. It correlates strongly with traditional concepts of "intelligence" or IQ.

Many scientists, mathematicians, engineers, doctors and economists function in this type of intelligence.

Naturalistic

This area has to do with nature, nurturing and relating information to one's natural surroundings. This type of intelligence was not part of Gardner's original theory of Multiple Intelligences, but was added to the theory in 1997. Those with it are said to have greater sensitivity to nature and their place within it, the ability to nurture and grow things, and greater ease in caring for, taming and interacting with animals. They may also be able to discern changes in weather or similar fluctuations in their natural surroundings. Recognizing and classifying things are at the core of a naturalist. They must connect a new experience with prior knowledge to truly learn something new.

"Naturalists" learn best when the subject involves collecting and analyzing, or is closely related to something prominent in nature; they also don't enjoy learning unfamiliar or seemingly useless subjects with little or no connections to nature. It is advised that naturalistic learners would learn more through being outside or in a kinesthetic way.

The theory behind this intelligence is often criticized, much like the spiritual or existential intelligence, as it is seen by many as not indicative of an intelligence but rather an interest.

Careers that suit those with this intelligence include scientists, naturalists, conservationists, gardeners and farmers.

Intrapersonal

This area has to do with introspective and self-reflective capacities. Those who are strongest in this intelligence are typically introverts and prefer to work alone. They are usually highly self-aware and capable of understanding their own emotions, goals and motivations. They often have an affinity for thought-based pursuits such as philosophy. They learn best when allowed to concentrate on the subject by themselves. There is often a high level of perfectionism associated with this intelligence.

Careers that suit those with this intelligence include philosophers, psychologists, theologians, writers and scientists.

Visual-spatial

This area has to do with vision and spatial judgment. People with strong visual-spatial intelligence are typically very good at visualizing and mentally manipulating objects. Those with strong spatial intelligence are often proficient at solving puzzles. They have a strong visual memory and are often artistically inclined. Those with visual-spatial intelligence also generally have a very good sense of direction and may also have very good hand-eye coordination, although this is normally seen as a characteristic of the bodily-kinesthetic intelligence.

Some critics point out the high correlation between the spatial and mathematical abilities, which seems to disprove the clear separation of the intelligences as Gardner theorized. Since solving a mathematical problem involves reassuringly manipulating symbols and numbers, spatial intelligence is involved in visually changing the reality. A thorough understanding of the two intelligences precludes this criticism, however, as the two intelligences do not precisely conform to the definitions of visual and mathematical abilities. Although they may share certain characteristics, they are easily distinguished by several factors, and there are many with strong logical-mathematical intelligence.

Careers that suit those with this intelligence include artists, engineers, and architects.

Musical

This area has to do with rhythm, music, and hearing. Those who have a high level of musical-rhythmic intelligence display greater sensitivity to sounds, rhythms, tones, and music. They normally have good pitch and may even have absolute pitch, and are able to sing, play musical instruments, and compose music. Since there is a strong auditory component to this intelligence, those who are strongest in it may learn best via lecture. In addition, they will often use songs or rhythms to learn and memorize information, and may work best with music playing in the background.

Careers that suit those with this intelligence include instrumentalists, singers, conductors, disc-jockeys, orators, writers (to a certain extent) and composers and sales reps.

Constancy of IQ

Intelligence Quotient

An **intelligence quotient** or **IQ** is a score derived from one of several different standardized tests attempting to measure intelligence. The term "IQ," borrowed from the German *Intelligenz-Quotient*, was coined by the German psychologist William Stern in 1912 as a proposed method of scoring early modern children's intelligence tests such as those developed by Alfred Binet and Theodore Simon in the early 20th Century. Although the term "IQ" is still in common use, the scoring of modern IQ tests such as the Wechsler Adult Intelligence Scale is now based on a projection of the subject's measured rank on the Gaussian bell curve with a centre value (average IQ) of 100, and a standard deviation of 15, although different tests may have different standard deviations. IQ scores have been shown to be associated with such factors as morbidity and mortality, parental social status, and to a substantial degree, parental IQ. While its inheritance has been investigated for nearly a century, controversy remains as to how much is inheritable, and the mechanisms of inheritance are still a matter of some debate.

IQ scores are used in many contexts: as predictors of educational achievement or special needs, by social scientists who study the distribution of IQ scores in populations and the relationships between IQ score and other variables, and as predictors of job performance and income.

The average IQ scores for many populations have been rising at an average rate of three points per decade since the early 20th century with most of the increase in the lower half of the IQ range: a phenomenon called the Flynn effect. It is disputed whether these changes in scores reflect real changes in intellectual abilities, or merely methodological problems with past or present testing.

IQ and the Brain

In 2004, Richard Haier, professor of psychology in the Department of Pediatrics and colleagues at University of California, Irvine and the University of New Mexico used MRI to obtain structural images of the brain in 47 normal adults who also took standard IQ tests. The study demonstrated that general human intelligence appears to be based on the volume and location of gray matter tissue in the brain also demonstrated that, of the brain's gray matter, only about 6 percent appeared to be related to IQ.

Many different sources of information have converged on the view that the frontal lobes are critical for fluid intelligence. Patients with damage to the frontal lobe are impaired on fluid intelligence tests (Duncan et al. 1995). The volume of frontal grey (Thompson et al. 2001) and white matter (Schoenemann et al. 2005) have also been associated with general intelligence. In addition, recent neuroimaging studies have limited this association to the lateral prefrontal cortex. Duncan and colleagues (2000) showed using Positron Emission Tomography that problem-solving tasks that correlated more highly with IQ also activate the lateral prefrontal cortex. More recently, Gray and colleagues (2003) used functional magnetic resonance imaging (fMRI) to show that those individuals that were more adept at resisting distraction on a demanding working memory task had both a higher IQ and increased prefrontal activity.

A study involving 307 children (age between six to nineteen) measuring the size of brain structures using magnetic resonance imaging (MRI) and measuring verbal and non-verbal abilities has been conducted (Shaw et al. 2006). The study has indicated that there is a relationship between IQ and the structure of the cortex—the characteristic change being the group with the superior IQ scores starts with thinner cortex in the early age then becomes thicker than average by the late teens.

There is "a highly significant association" between the CHRM2 gene and intelligence according to a 2006 Dutch family study. The study concluded that there was an association between the CHRM2 gene on chromosome 7 and Performance IQ, as measured by the Wechsler Adult Intelligence Scale-Revised. The Dutch family study used a sample of 667 individuals from 304 families. A similar association was found independently in the *Minnesota Twin and Family Study* (Comings et al. 2003) and by the Department of Psychiatry at the Washington University.

Significant injuries isolated to one side of the brain, especially those occurring at a young age, may not significantly affect IQ.

Studies reach conflicting conclusions regarding the controversial idea that brain size correlates positively with IQ. Jensen and Reed claim no direct correlation exists in nonpathological subjects. A more recent meta-analysis suggests otherwise.

An alternative approach has sought to link differences in neural plasticity with intelligence, and this view has recently received some empirical support.

Assessment of Intelligence

On the dawn of the second century of scientific-based mental testing, the intelligence is viewed as a diffuse notion with a great number of theories, attempting to explain it. There's no universal definition of what intelligence is and that's why each of them tend to explain it in its own way. A commonly accepted definition is by Boring (1923), stating that "intelligence is what is measured by intelligence tests", or I would say, it is what they try to measure. What is important for this essay is that the subject measured by intelligence tests is a variety of cognitive abilities (semantic relations, general reasoning, sensorimotor functioning, spatial orientation, etc.), with the values behind the intelligence term tending to express the overall score.

The Uses of Intelligence Tests

Lewis M. Terman (1916)

Intelligence tests of retarded school children. Numerous studies of the age-grade progress of school children have afforded convincing evidence of the magnitude and seriousness of the retardation problem. Statistics collected in hundreds of cities in the United States show that between a third and a half of the school children fail to progress through the grades at the expected rate; that from 10 to 15 per cent are retarded two years or more; and that from 5 to 8 per cent are retarded at least three years. More than 10 per cent of the $400,000,000 annually expended in the United States for school instruction is devoted to re-teaching children what they have already been taught but have failed to learn.

The first efforts at reform which resulted from these findings were based on the supposition that the evils which had been discovered could be remedied by the individualizing of instruction, by improved methods of promotion, by increased attention to children's health, and by other reforms in school administration. Although reforms along these lines have been productive of much good, they have nevertheless been in a measure disappointing. The trouble was, they were too often based upon the assumption that under the right conditions all children would be equally, or almost equally, capable of making satisfactory school progress. Psychological studies of school children by means of standardized intelligence tests have shown that this supposition is not in accord with the facts. It has been found that children do not fall into two well-defined groups, the "feeble-minded" and the "normal." Instead, there are many grades of intelligence, ranging from idiocy on the one hand to genius on the other. Among those classed as normal, vast individual differences have been found to exist in original mental endowment, differences which affect profoundly the capacity to profit from school instruction. We are beginning to realize that the school must take into account, more seriously than it has yet done, the existence and significance of these differences in endowment. Instead of wasting energy in the vain attempt to hold mentally slow and defective children up to a level of progress which is normal to the average child, it will be wiser to take account of the inequalities of children in original endowment and to differentiate the course of study in such a way that each child will be allowed to progress at the rate which is normal to him, whether that rate be rapid or slow.

While we cannot hold all children to the same standard of school progress, we can at least prevent the kind of retardation which involves failure and the repetition of a school grade. It is well enough recognized that children do not enter with very much zest upon school work in which they have once failed. Failure crushes self-confidence and destroys the spirit of work. It is a sad fact that a large proportion of children in the schools are acquiring the habit of failure. The remedy, of course, is to measure out the work for each child in proportion to his mental ability.

Before an engineer constructs a railroad bridge or trestle, he studies the materials to be used, and learns by means of tests exactly the amount of strain per unit of size his materials will be able to withstand. He does not work empirically, and count upon patching up the mistakes which may later appear under the stress of actual use. The educational engineer should emulate this example. Tests and forethought must take the place of failure and patchwork. Our efforts have been too long directed by "trial and error." It is time to leave off guessing and to acquire a scientific knowledge of the material with which we have to deal. When instruction must be repeated, it means that the school, as well as the pupil, has failed.

Every child who fails in his school work or is in danger of failing should be given a mental examination. The examination takes less than one hour, and the result will contribute more to a real understanding of the case than anything else that could be done. It is necessary to determine whether a given child is unsuccessful in school because of poor native ability, or because of poor instruction, lack of interest, or some other removable cause.

It is not sufficient to establish any number of special classes, if they are to be made the dumping-ground for all kinds of troublesome cases — the feeble-minded, the physically defective, the merely backward, the truants, the incorrigibles, etc. Without scientific diagnosis and classification of these children the educational work of the special class must blunder along in the dark. In such diagnosis and classification our main reliance must always be in mental tests, properly used and properly interpreted.

Intelligence tests of the feeble-minded: Thus far intelligence tests have found their chief application in the identification and grading of the feeble-minded. Their value for this purpose is twofold. In the first place, it is necessary to ascertain the degree of defect before it is possible to decide intelligently upon either the content or the method of instruction suited to the training of the backward child. In the second place, intelligence tests are rapidly extending our conception of "feeble-mindedness" to include milder degrees of defect than have generally been associated with this term. The earlier methods of diagnosis caused a majority of the higher grade defectives to be overlooked. Previous to the development of psychological methods the low-grade moron was about as high a type of defective as most physicians or even psychologists were able to identify as feeble-minded.

Wherever intelligence tests have been made in any considerable number in the schools, they have shown that not far from 2 per cent of the children enrolled have a grade of intelligence which, however long they live, will never develop beyond the level which is normal to the average child of 11 or 12 years. The large majority of these belong to the moron grade; that is, their mental development will stop somewhere between the 7-year and 12-year level of intelligence, more often between 9 and 12.

The more we learn about such children, the clearer it becomes that they must be looked upon as real defectives. They may be able to drag along to the fourth, fifth, or sixth grades, but even by the age of 16 or 18 years they are never able to cope successfully with the more abstract and difficult parts of the common-school course of study. They may master a certain amount of rote learning, such as that involved in reading and in the manipulation of number combinations, but they cannot be taught to meet new conditions effectively or to think, reason, and judge as normal persons do.

It is safe to predict that in the near future intelligence tests will bring tens of thousands of these high-grade defectives under the surveillance and protection of society. This will ultimately result in curtailing the reproduction of feeble-mindedness and in the elimination of an enormous amount of crime, pauperism, and industrial inefficiency. It is hardly necessary to emphasize that the high-grade cases, of the type now so frequently overlooked, are precisely the ones whose guardianship it is most important for the State to assume.

Intelligence tests of delinquents: One of the most important facts brought to light by the use of intelligence tests is the frequent association of delinquency and mental deficiency. Although it has long been recognized that the proportion of feeble-mindedness among offenders is rather large, the real amount has, until recently, been underestimated even by the most competent students of criminology.

Understanding and Enhancing the Creative Process with New Technologies

A simple but accurate review on this new Human-Computer Interactions (HCI) angle for promoting creativity has been written by Todd Lubart, an invitation full of creative ideas to develop further this new field.

Groupware and other Computer Supported Collaborative Work (CSCW) platforms are now the stage of Network Creativity on the web or on other private networks. These tools have made more obvious the existence of a more connective, cooperative and collective nature of creativity rather than the prevaling individual one. Creativity Research on Global Virtual Teams is showing that the creative process is affected by the national identities, cognitive and conative profiles, anonymous interactions at times and many other factors affecting the teams members, depending on the early or later stages of the cooperative creative process. They are also showing how NGO's cross cultural virtual team's innovation in Africa would also benefit from the pooling of best global practices online. Such tools enhancing cooperative creativity may have a great impact on society and as such should be tested while they are built following the Motto : "Build the Camera while shooting the film". Some European FP7 scientific programs like Paradiso are answering a need for advanced experimentally-driven research including large scale experimentation test-beds to discover the technical, societal, and economic implications of such groupware and collaborative tools to the Internet.

On the other hand Creativity research may one day be pooled with a computable Metalangguage like IEML from the University of Ottawa Collective Intelligence Chair, Pierre Levy. It might be a good tool to provide an interdisciplinary definition and a rather unified theory of creativity. The creative processes being highly fuzzy, the programming of cooperative tools for creativity and innovation should be adaptive and flexible. Empirical Modelling seems to be a good choice for Humanities Computing.

If all the activity of the universe could be traced with appropriate captors, it is likely that one could see the creative nature of the universe to which humans are active contributors. After the web of documents, the Web of Things might shed some light on such a universal creative phenomenon which should not be restricted to humans. In order to trace and enhance cooperative and collective creativity, Metis Reflexive Global Virtual Team has worked for the last few years on the development of a Trace Composer at the intersection of personal experience and social knowledge.

Metis Reflexive Team has also identified a paradigm for the study of creativity to bridge European theory of "useless" and non instrumentalized creativity, North American more pragmatic creativity and Chinese culture stressing more creativity as a holistic process of continuity rather than radical change and originality. This paradigm is mostly based on the work of the German philosopher Hans Joas, one that emphasizes the creative character of human action. This model allows also for a more comprehensive theory of action. Joas elaborates some implications of his model for theories of social movements and social change. The connexion between concepts like creation, innovation, production and expression is facilitated by the creativity of action as a metaphore but also as scientific concept.

The Creativity and Cognition conference series, sponsored by the ACM and running since 1993 has been an important venue for publishing research on the intersection between technology and creativity. The conference now runs biannually, next taking place in 2009.

The Process of Creativity-So what is creativity and what is the mechanism through which people actually create new ideas, solutions or concepts? According to many theorists, creativity is about chance or serendipity or making discoveries by 'accident'. So the creative process, according to this explanation is an 'accident'. This means that while you're trying out several methods, a best method or a solution to your problem arises out of nowhere and by chance you discover something totally unique. Some people would suggest that the creative process is more of trying to find out new relations between older known concepts so this is less about originality and more about 'experience'. The more experienced you are in a particular subject area, the more likely you are to consider creative solutions. Creativity has also been described as a moment of 'insight'. It is almost like enlightenment and divine intervention and a flash and the trick is to prolong this moment and creative individuals are people who can develop their sudden insights. So the creative process can be about a sudden chance, novel use of the knowledge/ experience or a sudden insight. The creative process thus involves using several possibilities/ methods and past experiences to arrive at sudden solutions through insights or accidents.

In 1926, Graham Wallas described stages of creativity in which a creative idea is first prepared, then internalized through incubation, after which the creative individual uses the illumination or insight to finally go through the verification process of applying the idea. Psychologist JP Guilford explained creativity with his concept of convergent and divergent thinking and convergent thinking is about trying to find the single correct solution to a problem and divergent thinking is the generation of multiple creative solutions to a problem. Creativity is thus characterized by divergent thinking and generation of multiple possibilities. According to the Geneplore model developed by Finke, Ward and Smith (1992), creativity involves two phases-the generative phase in which the individual generates constructs from pre-inventive structures or known processes/ideas and the exploratory phase in which pre-inventive structures are interpreted to come up with new creative ideas. Most of these psychological theories seem to be emphasizing on preexisting mental structures through knowledge and experience and using these structures for novel or unique solutions. The creative process is thus all about insight, 'a sudden flash', almost like a moment of realization and it has been described as serendipity or divine intervention by scientists and artists alike who have tried to described their moment of discovery, although the role of previous knowledge and experience is an equally important background factor. The scientists and artists are able to realize the potential of these 'flashes' and are able to recognize, capture and prolong their moments of insight for better realization of their creative goals.

Why is it Easier to Measure Intelligence than Creativity?

To be intelligent one has or shows understanding, is clever and quick of mind, whereas to be creative is to bring something into existence, to give rise to something or to originate. It seems easier to assess levels of intelligence, through the use of IQ tests than it is to assess levels of creativity as there is no such equivalent test.

IQ tests usually select an activity or skill and then design tests to measure individual performances in the specified activity. A high score will indicate a high level of performance and a low score will indicate a low level of performance. However it is difficult to measure creativity in such a way because the skills are harder to define as they are usually unique and diverse.

"Divergent thinking" tests of "creativity" were designed without any substantial validation. They differ from "convergent" tests of "intelligence" in that they are open ended and do not have right or wrong answers. There are also problems in validating creativity because it is very difficult to define what terms such as "giftedness" and "genius" mean.

There is an apparent contradiction between the predictability of objective tests and the unpredictability of creativity. Confusion arises with the measurement of general and specific intellectual skills as there is no clear idea about how they interact together in creativity. The Life Cycle affects measurements too as IQ-related skills and knowledge improve with age until adulthood, whereas creativity seems to occur randomly at different ages. It seems impossible to measure creativity unless it depends on a non creative, intellectual skill. On the other hand intelligence is relatively easy to assess through IQ tests, which give clear indications of levels of performance.

The Process of Creativity

Creativity is a mental and social process involving the generation of new ideas or concepts, or new associations of the creative mind between existing ideas or concepts. Creativity is fuelled by the process of either conscious or unconscious insight. An alternative conception of creativeness is that it is simply the act of making something new.

From a scientific point of view, the products of creative thought (sometimes referred to as divergent thought) are usually considered to have both originality *and* appropriateness.

Although intuitively a simple phenomenon, it is in fact quite complex. It has been studied from the perspectives of behavioural psychology, social psychology, psychometrics, cognitive science, artificial intelligence, philosophy, history, economics, design research, business, and management, among others. The studies have covered everyday creativity, exceptional creativity and even artificial creativity. Unlike many phenomena in science, there is no single, authoritative perspective or definition of creativity. And unlike many phenomena in psychology, there is no standardized measurement technique. Creativity has been attributed variously to divine intervention, cognitive processes, the social environment, personality traits, and chance ("accident", "serendipity"). It has been associated with genius, mental illness and humour. Some say it is a trait we are born with; others say it can be taught with the application of simple techniques. Creativity has also been viewed as a beneficence of a muse or Muses.

Although popularly associated with art and literature, it is also an essential part of innovation and invention and is important in professions such as business, economics, architecture, industrial design, graphic design, advertising, music, science and engineering.

Despite, or perhaps because of, the ambiguity and multi-dimensional nature of creativity, entire industries have been spawned from the pursuit of creative ideas and the development of creativity techniques.

Creativity has been associated with right or forehead brain activity or even specifically with lateral thinking.

Some students of creativity have emphasized an element of chance in the creative process. Linus Pauling, asked at a public lecture how one creates scientific theories, replied that one must endeavour to come up with *many* ideas — then discard the useless ones.

Another adequate definition of creativity is that it is an "assumptions-breaking process." Creative ideas are often generated when one discards preconceived assumptions and attempts a new approach or method that might seem to others unthinkable.

Creativity and Intelligence

There has been debate in the psychological literature about whether intelligence and creativity are part of the same process (the conjoint hypothesis) or represent distinct mental processes (the disjoint hypothesis). Evidence from attempts to look at correlations between intelligence and creativity from the 1950s onwards, by authors such as Barron, Guilford or Wallach and

Kogan, regularly suggested that correlations between these concepts were low enough to justify treating them as distinct concepts.

Some researchers believe that creativity is the outcome of the same cognitive processes as intelligence, and is only judged as creativity in terms of its consequences, i.e. when the outcome of cognitive processes happens to produce something novel, a view which Perkins has termed the "nothing special" hypothesis.

A very popular model is what has come to be known as "the threshold hypothesis", proposed by Ellis Paul Torrance, which holds that a high degree of intelligence appears to be a necessary but not sufficient condition for high creativity. This means that, in a general sample, there will be a positive correlation between creativity and intelligence, but this correlation will not be found if only a sample of the most highly intelligent people are assessed. Research into the threshold hypothesis, however, has produced mixed results ranging from enthusiastic support to refutation and rejection.

An alternative perspective, Renzulli's three-rings hypothesis, sees giftedness as based on both intelligence and creativity. More on both the threshold hypothesis and Renzulli's work can be found in O'Hara and Sternberg.

Kinds of intelligent performance that matter in everyday life, such as social intelligence.

Most of theories of multiple intelligences are relatively recent in origin, though Louis Thurstone proposed a theory of multiple "primary abilities" in the early 20th Century.

Triarchic Theory of Intelligence

Robert Sternberg's triarchic theory of intelligence proposes three fundamental aspects of intelligence — analytic, creative, and practical — of which only the first is measured to any significant extent by mainstream tests. His investigations suggest the need for a balance between analytic intelligence, on the one hand, and creative and especially practical intelligence on the other.

Emotional Intelligence

Daniel Goleman and several other researchers have developed the concept of emotional intelligence and claim it is at least as "important" as more traditional sorts of intelligence. These theories grew from observations of human development and of brain injury victims who demonstrate an acute loss of a particular cognitive function — e.g. the ability to think numerically, or the ability to understand written language — without showing any loss in other cognitive areas.

Empirical Evidence

IQ proponents have pointed out that IQ's predictive validity has been repeatedly demonstrated, for example in predicting important non-academic outcomes such as job performance (see IQ), whereas the various multiple intelligence theories have little or no such support. Meanwhile, the relevance and even the existence of multiple intelligences have not been borne out when actually tested. A set of ability tests that do not correlate together would support the claim that multiple intelligences are independent of each other.

Factors Affecting Intelligence

Intelligence is an ill-defined, difficult to quantify concept. Accordingly, the IQ tests used to measure intelligence provide only approximations of the posited 'real' intelligence. In addition, a number of theoretically unrelated properties are known to correlate with IQ such as race, gender and height but since correlation does not imply causation the true relationship between these factors is uncertain. Factors affecting IQ may be divided into biological and environmental.

Biological

Evidence suggests that genetic variation has a significant impact on IQ, accounting for three fourths in adults. Despite the high heritability of IQ, few genes have been found to have a substantial effect on IQ, suggesting that IQ is the product of interaction between multiple genes.

Other biological factors correlating with IQ include ratio of brain weight to body weight and the volume and location of gray matter tissue in the brain. Because intelligence appears to be at least partly dependent on brain structure and the genes shaping brain development, it has been proposed that genetic engineering could be used to enhance the intelligence of animals, a process sometimes called biological uplift in science fiction.

Experiments on mice have demonstrated superior ability in learning and memory in various behavioural tasks.

Environmental

Evidence suggests that family environmental factors may have an effect upon childhood IQ, accounting for up to a quarter of the variance. On the other hand, by late adolescence this correlation disappears, such that adoptive siblings are no more similar in IQ than strangers. Moreover, adoption studies indicate that, by adulthood, adoptive siblings are no more similar in IQ than strangers, while twins and full siblings show an IQ correlation.

Consequently, in the context of the nature versus nurture debate, the "nature" component appears to be much more important than the "nurture" component in explaining IQ variance in the general population.

There are indications that, in middle age, intelligence is influenced by life style choices (e.g., long working hours).

Cultural factors also play a role in intelligence. For example, on a sorting task to measure intelligence, Westerners tend to take a taxonomic approach while the Kpelle people take a more functional approach.

For example, instead of grouping food and tools into separate categories, a Kpelle participant stated "the knife goes with the orange because it cuts it"

Ethical Issues

Since intelligence is susceptible to modification through the manipulation of environment, the ability to influence intelligence raises ethical issues. Transhumanist theorists study the possibilities and consequences of developing and using techniques to enhance human abilities and aptitudes, and ameliorate what it regards as undesirable and unnecessary aspects of the human condition; eugenics is a social philosophy which advocates the improvement of human hereditary traits through various forms of intervention.

The perception of eugenics has varied throughout history, from a social responsibility required of society, to an immoral, racist stance.

Neuroethics considers the ethical, legal and social implications of neuroscience, and deals with issues such as difference between treating a human neurological disease and enhancing the human brain, and how wealth impacts access to neurotechnology. Neuroethical issues interact with the ethics of human genetic engineering.

Identification and Promotion of Creativity

Creativity is the condition for innovation.

Creativity without realization, an idea without implemention has no effect.

Creativity and innovation are essential factors for companies to succeed in business.

But how do you get to a genious idea and how can you proceed from there to innovation and finally to realization?

This forum shall activate your creative potential and shall give you incentives, information about techniques, methodologies, etc., and finally also a view at the human factor in this area.

Creativity, innovation, and initiative are psychological processes that facilitate the transformation of individual work roles, teams, and organisations into desired future states. Therefore, the present paper focuses on potential research trends in this increasingly important area.

Specifically, we identify three substantive gaps reflecting the needs for greater process differentiation, concept integration, and cross-cultural analysis. First, potential differential antecedents of specific creativity or innovation phases have received insufficient attention. Second, the creativity and innovation research domain may benefit from an integration of recently developed proactivity concepts such as personal initiative and voice behaviour. Third, cross-cultural differences in values, motivational orientations, and leadership preferences may determine how creativity and innovation are enacted and cultivated across the globe. With respect to each of these future challenges, we provide suggestions for theoretical and empirical advancements and discuss potential practical and methodological developments.

Thinking—Convergent and Divergent Thinking

Thinking Styles

Hudson (1967) studied English schoolboys, and found that conventional measures of intelligence did not always do justice to their abilities. The tests gave credit for problem-solving which produced the "right" answer, but under-estimated creativity and unconventional approaches to problems. He concluded that there were two different forms of thinking or ability in play here:

- One he called "convergent" thinking, in which the person is good at bringing material from a variety of sources to bear on a problem, in such a way as to produce the "correct" answer. This kind of thinking is particularly appropriate in science, maths and technology.
- Because of the need for consistency and reliability, this is really the only form of thinking which standardised intelligence tests, (and even national exams) can test
- The other he termed "divergent" thinking. Here the student's skill is in broadly creative elaboration of ideas prompted by a stimulus, and is more suited to artistic pursuits and study in the humanities.
- In order to get at this kind of thinking, he devised open-ended tests, such as the "Uses of Objects" test

Convergent and Divergent Production

Convergent and **divergent production** are the two types of human response to a set problem that were identified by

J. P. Guilford. Guilford observed that most individuals display a preference for either convergent or divergent thinking. (Others observe that most people prefer a convergent closure). As opposed to say TRIZ or Lateral Thinking divergent thinking is **not about tools** for creativity or thinking, but a way of categorizing what can be observed.

Divergent Thinking

According to Guilford College, divergent or synthetic thinking is the ability to draw on ideas from across disciplines and fields of inquiry to reach a deeper understanding of the world and one's place in it.

There is a movement in education that maintains divergent thinking might create more resourceful students. Rather than presenting a series of problems for rote memorization or resolution, divergent thinking presents open-ended problems and encourages students to develop their own solutions to problems.

Divergent production is the creative generation of multiple answers to a set problem. For example, *find uses for 1 meter lengths of black cotton.*

Convergent Thinking

Convergent thinking is oriented towards deriving the single best (or correct) answer to a clearly defined question. It emphasizes speed, accuracy, logic, and the like, and focuses on accumulating information, recognizing the familiar, reapplying set techniques, and preserving the already known. It is based on familiarity with what is already known (i.e., knowledge), and is most effective in situations where a ready-made answer exists and needs simply to be recalled from stored information, or worked out from what is already known by applying conventional and logical search, recognition and decision-making strategies. (OWAIS)

Use and Implementations

The terms Divergent/Convergent thinking is widely used to **describe** a creative development process.

In some "schools" the model is even used for facilitation of meetings etc. many facilitators and leaders thus seek to end any facilitation with convergent thinking.

Critic of the Analytic/dialectic Approach

While the observations made in psychology can be used to analyze the thinking of humans, such categories may also lead to oversimplifications and dialectic thinking.

The systematic use of convergent thinking may well lead to what is known as Group think-thus one should probably combine systematic use with critical thinking.

Categorizing thinkers as "divergent" or "convergent" may seem appropriate for the purpose of general analyzes.

Unit-VII

Motivation and Group Dynamics

Motivation and Learning

Basic principles of motivation exist that are applicable to learning in any situation.

1. The environment can be used to focus the student's attention on what needs to be learned.

   Teachers who create warm and accepting yet businesslike atmospheres will promote persistent effort and favourable attitudes toward learning. This strategy will be successful in children and in adults. Interesting visual aids, such as booklets, posters, or practice equipment, motivate learners by capturing their attention and curiosity.

2. Incentives motivate learning.

   Incentives include privileges and receiving praise from the instructor. The instructor determines an incentive that is likely to motivate an individual at a particular time. In a general learning situation, self-motivation without rewards will not succeed. Students must find satisfaction in learning based on the understanding that the goals are useful to them or, less commonly, based on the pure enjoyment of exploring new things.

3. Internal motivation is longer lasting and more self-directive than is external motivation, which must be repeatedly reinforced by praise or concrete rewards.

Some individuals — particularly children of certain ages and some adults — have little capacity for internal motivation and must be guided and reinforced constantly. The use of incentives is based on the principle that learning occurs more effectively when the student experiences feelings of satisfaction. Caution should be exercised in using external rewards when they are not absolutely necessary. Their use may be followed by a decline in internal motivation.

4. Learning is most effective when an individual is ready to learn, that is, when one wants to know something.

   Sometimes the student's readiness to learn comes with time, and the instructor's role is to encourage its development. If a desired change in behaviour is urgent, the instructor may need to supervised directly to ensure that the desired behaviour occurs. If a student is not *ready to learn,* he or she may not be reliable in following instructions and therefore must be supervised and have the instructions repeated again and again.

5. Motivation is enhanced by the way in which the instructional material is organized.

   In general, the best organized material makes the information meaningful to the individual. One method of organization includes relating new tasks to those already known. Other ways to relay meaning are to determine whether the persons being taught understand the final outcome desired and instruct them to compare and contrast ideas.

None of the techniques will produce sustained motivation unless the goals are realistic for the learner. The basic learning principle involved is that *success is more predictably motivating than is failure.* Ordinarily, people will choose activities of intermediate uncertainty rather than those that are difficult (little likelihood of success) or easy (high probability of success). For goals of high value there is less tendency to choose more difficult conditions. Having learners assist in defining goals increases the probability that they will understand them and want to reach them. However, students sometimes have unrealistic notions about what they can accomplish. Possibly they do not understand the precision with which a skill must be carried out or have the depth of knowledge to master some material. To identify realistic goals, instructors must be skilled in assessing a student's readiness or a student's progress toward goals.

1. Because learning requires changed in beliefs and behaviour, it normally produces a mild level of anxiety.

   This is useful in motivating the individual. However, severe anxiety is incapacitating. A high degree of stress is inherent in some educational situations. If anxiety is severe, the individual's perception of what is going on around him or her is limited. Instructors must be able to identify anxiety and understand its effect on learning. They also have a responsibility to avoid causing severe anxiety in learners by setting ambiguous of unrealistically high goals for them.

2. It is important to help each student set goals and to provide informative feedback regarding progress toward the goals.

   Setting a goal demonstrates an intention to achieve and activates learning from one day to the next. It also directs the student's activities toward the goal and offers an opportunity to experience success.

3. Both affiliation and approval are strong motivators.

   People seek others with whom to compare their abilities, opinions, and emotions. Affiliation can also result in direct anxiety reduction by the social acceptance and the mere presence of others. However, these motivators can also lead to conformity, competition, and other behaviours that may seem as negative.

4. Many behaviours result from a combination of motives.

   It is recognized that no grand theory of motivation exists. However, motivation is so necessary for learning that strategies should be planned to organize a continuous and interactive motivational dynamic for maximum effectiveness. The general principles of motivation are interrelated. A single teaching action can use many of them simultaneously.

Finally, it should be said that an enormous gap exists between knowing that learning must be motivated and identifying the specific motivational components of any particular act. Instructors must focus on learning patterns of motivation for an individual or group, with the realization that errors will be common.

Kind of Motives

A MOTIVE may be defined as meaning that which acts as an inducement to preference or choice. 'In other words it is a very strong influence toward some object to be attained.

Just what these influences are depends entirely upon the nature of the person and on the object to be attained. We often hear the expression, and doubtless use it as often ourselves, "What was your motive in doing this?" meaning what caused you or what influenced you to act in such a manner. We may state with truth that every wilful act has its inducement or cause. Just as in mathematics there is a reason for every step, so also in every act there is a motive or cause. From the child on up the individual can give a reason for each and every one of his voluntary acts however small and mean the reason may be. Still it is a reason. It may only be a certain state of consciousness which happens to be uppermost in a man's mind as he acts.

Very often Intention and Motive are confused; in fact they are used interchangeably in society. Notwithstanding this fact there is a vast difference in their meaning. Intention is what a man means to do, while Motive is the personal frame of mind which indicates why he means to do it. Therefore Intention has the stronger moral value, while Motive renders the consequences interesting and attractive. Motive is that which makes the difference between one act and another.

As we now know the difference between Intention and Motive, let us examine the different kinds of Motives. Motive may be divided into two classes, Egoistical and Altruistical. Both classes are absolutely necessary in our daily life. Let us first look at egoistic motives or the ones which concern the self only. Our original instincts are such that their objects are to look after the advantages of the self. However everything depends upon the sort of self maintained. What would become of a person if he would not struggle for food and strive against obstacles? What would become of society? Self-preserving instincts must be therefore socially conservative. No one has a right to neglect his own interests, hoping some one else will care for them. The man who takes exercise because he thinks of his health must be commanded, but the one who is thinking continually of his health and excludes other thoughts must be condemned.

Theories of Motivation

Ever wonder why some people seem to be very successful, highly motivated individuals? Where does the energy, the drive, or the direction come from? Motivation is an area of psychology that has gotten a great deal of attention, especially in the recent years. The reason is because we all want to be successful, we all want direction and drive, and we all want to be seen as motivated. There are several distinct theories of motivation we will discuss in this section. Some include basic biological forces, while others seem to transcend concrete explanation. Let's talk about the five major theories of motivation.

Instinct Theory

Instinct theory is derived from our biological make-up. We've all seen spider's webs and perhaps even witnessed a spider in the tedious job of creating its home and trap. We've all seen birds in their nests, feeding their young or painstakingly placing the twigs in place to form their new home. How do spiders know how to spin webs? How do birds now how to build nests?

The answer is biology. All creatures are born with specific innate knowledge about how to survive. Animals are born with the capacity and often times knowledge of how to survive by spinning webs, building nests, avoiding danger, and reproducing. These innate tendencies are preprogrammed at birth, they are in our genes, and even if the spider never saw a web before, never witnessed its creation, it would still know how to create one. Humans have the same types of innate tendencies. Babies are born with a unique ability that allows them to survive; they are born with the ability to cry. Without this, how would others know when to feed the baby, know when he needed changing, or when she wanted attention and affection? Crying allows a human infant to survive. We are also born with particular reflexes which promote survival. The most important of these include sucking, swallowing, coughing, blinking. Newborns can perform physical movements to avoid pain; they will turn their head if touched on their cheek and search for a nipple (rooting reflex); and they will grasp an object that touches the palm of their hands.

Drive Reduction Theory

According to Clark Hull (1943, 1952), humans have internal biological needs which motivate us to perform a certain way. These needs, or drives, are defined by Hull as internal states of arousal or tension which must be reduced. A prime example would be the internal feelings of hunger or thirst, which motivates us to eat. According to this theory, we are driven to reduce these drives so that we may maintain a sense of internal calmness.

Arousal Theory

Similar to Hull's Drive Reduction Theory, Arousal theory states that we are driven to maintain a certain level of arousal in order to feel comfortable. Arousal refers to a state of emotional, intellectual, and physical activity. It is different from the above theory, however, because it doesn't rely on only a reduction of tension, but a balanced amount. It also does better to explain why people climb mountains, go to school, or watch sad movies.

Psychoanalytic Theory

Remember Sigmund Freud and his five part theory of personality. As part of this theory, he believed that humans have only two basic drives: Eros and Thanatos, or the Life and

Death drives. According to Psychoanalytic theory, everything we do, every thought we have, and every emotion we experience has one of two goals: to help us survive or to prevent our destruction. This is similar to instinct theory, however, Freud believed that the vast majority of our knowledge about these drives is buried in the unconscious part of the mind.

Psychoanalytic theory therefore argues that we go to school because it will help assure our survival in terms of improved finances, more money for healthcare, or even an improved ability to find a spouse. We move to better school districts to improve our children's ability to survive and continue our family tree. We demand safety in our cars, toys, and in our homes. We want criminal locked away, and we want to be protected against poisons, terrorists, and any thing else that could lead to our destruction. According to this theory, everything we do, everything we are can be traced back to the two basic drives

Humanistic Theory

Although discussed last, humanistic theory is perhaps the most well know theory of motivation. According to this theory, humans are driven to achieve their maximum potential and will always do so unless obstacles are placed in their way. These obstacles include hunger, thirst, financial problems, safety issues, or anything else that takes our focus away from maximum psychological growth.

The best way to describe this theory is to utilize the famous pyramid developed by Abraham Maslow (1970) called the Hierarchy of Needs. Maslow believed that humans have specific needs that must be met and that if lower level needs go unmet, we can not possible strive for higher level needs. The Hierarchy of Needs shows that at the lower level, we must focus on basic issues such as food, sleep, and safety. Without food, without sleep, how could we possible focus on the higher level needs such as respect, education, and recognition?

Maslow's Hierarchy of Needs

Maslow's hierarchy of needs is a theory in psychology, proposed by Abraham Maslow in his 1943 paper *A Theory of*

Human Motivation, which he subsequently extended to include his observations of humans' innate curiosity.

Maslow studied what he called exemplary people such as Albert Einstein, Jane Addams, Eleanor Roosevelt, and Frederick Douglass rather than mentally ill or neurotic people, writing that "the study of crippled, stunted, immature, and unhealthy specimens can yield only a cripple psychology and a cripple philosophy." Maslow also studied the healthiest one percent of the college student population. In his book, *The Farther Reaches of Human Nature*, Maslow writes, "By ordinary standards of this kind of laboratory research... this simply was not research at all. My generalizations grew out of my selection of certain kinds of people. Obviously, other judges are needed."

Representations

Maslow's hierarchy of needs is predetermined in order of importance. It is often depicted as a pyramid consisting of five levels: the first lower level is being associated with physiological needs, while the top levels are termed growth needs associated with psychological needs. Deficiency needs must be met first. Once these are met, seeking to satisfy growth needs drives personal growth. The higher needs in this hierarchy only come into focus when the lower needs in the pyramid are met. Once an individual has moved upwards to the next level, needs in the lower level will no longer be prioritized. If a lower set of needs is no longer being met, the individual will temporarily re-prioritize those needs by focusing attention on the unfulfilled needs, but will not permanently regress to the lower level. For instance, a businessman at the esteem level who is diagnosed with cancer will spend a great deal of time concentrating on his health (physiological needs), but will continue to value his work performance (esteem needs) and will likely return to work during periods of remission.

Role of Rewards and Punishments

Rewards

Rewards can serve as effective incentives—if the person is interested in the reward. School grades are a case in point. The reward of a good grade is important to some students--but of no interest to others. A reason why some students exert little effort for grades is that—to use Dr William Glasser's vocabulary—grades are not in their "Quality World." If a good grade or any reward is not important to the person, it has little value as an incentive.

Rewards can also serve as wonderful acknowledgements—ways of congratulating merit and demonstrating appreciation. Student of the week or employee of the month are examples of such acknowledgements. But notice that these are awarded after the behaviour—not as bribes beforehand.

As opposed to using rewards as incentives and acknowledgements, giving rewards for expected standards of behaviour is counterproductive. It is also based on the outmoded idea that all behaviour is modified thorough external approaches, similar to the techniques used to train animals. Internal approaches—such as self-talk—have no place in this mindset.

People who use this behavioral approach—often referred to as behaviour modification—have just one objective: changing behaviour. Practitioners of this approach do NOT promote ADULT values. By rewarding kids with something youngsters value (candy, stickers, prizes, etc.), we simply reinforce their CHILDHOOD values. In the process, we lose opportunities to pass on OUR values—such as generosity, kindness, responsibility, perseverance, and integrity. What we really hope to do is to teach young people about values that will last a lifetime. So, while most kids will do what you want them to do to get the treat, and it might look as if they are becoming more mature, they have not moved one step further towards becoming more responsible.

Punishments

No argument is presented here against such societal practices for adults who have been convicted of socially harmful behaviour. If you believe that an eight-year-old is an eighteen-yea-old, then it may seem natural to treat a young person with similar approaches. However, if you believe that young people are not yet adults, then the use of punishment to raise responsibility must be examined.

A common myth is that imposed punishments are necessary to change young people's behaviour. If this type of punishment worked, then once a youngster is punished the same behaviour would not be repeated. If you have used punishments to change behaviour and the same behaviour was repeated, read on.

Not too many of us remember that the horse pulling the buggy was urged on by a flick of the whip and that information was pounded into students by the cane, the strap, or fear of them. But since then, we have found better ways to teach; yet we are still using the horse and buggy approach to foster social responsibility in an era when both society and the nature of youth have dramatically changed.

Punishments operate on the theory young people must experience pain in order to grow into responsibility. We are expecting people whom we "intentionally hurt" to act constructively thereafter. But can you recall the last time you felt bad and did something good? People cannot think positively with negative feelings. People do "good" when they feel good. Imposed punishments can force compliance but never commitment. Have you ever seen anyone punished into commitment? Punishments kill the very thing we are attempting to do—change behaviour into something that is positive and socially appropriate.

One reason we keep thinking punishment works is that sometimes the behaviour stops. This may be the case with very young children if the behaviour is caught early before it becomes a habit and if the punishment itself is a novel experience. However, we must also consider whether or not the subject understands which action is being punished.

Punishments are ineffective with far too many young people. Escalation is a testament to its ineffectiveness. In schools when punishments fails to work, inevitably more punishments are prescribed, and the cycle perpetuates itself. By the time some students reach the secondary level, they have been talked to, lectured at, sent out of class, kept after school, referred to the office, referred to Saturday school, suspended in school, suspended from school—and they simply no longer care.

Punishments are temporary and transitory. Fear and force only produce changes in the short run. Once a punishment ends, the youngster has "served his time" and is "free and clear" from further responsibility. A coercive approach that works in the short run does not mean it is effective in the long run. Threatening a youngster with punishment may force compliance--but only so long as the threat is present. Needless to say, it does not change behaviour when the coercion is gone.

Level of Aspiration

BASUMALLIK AND BANERJEE, WEINSTEIN, AND RAY have reported findings from India, the United States, and Australia which call into question the once generally accepted relationship between high achievement motivation and intermediate levels of risk-preference (1). It now appears that the two variables are essentially unrelated. Wolk and Du Cette (2) also found no overall relationship but reported that when they studied only the "internals" (in Rotter's (3) sense) in their sample, the predicted relationship could be found quite strongly. Their work in this respect has been praised by Lefcourt (4), but it is nonetheless hard to see how there could be a strong relationship in one half of the sample, no relationship in the other half, and also no relationship overall. One would surely have thought that the overall relationship would be some sort of weaker (in-between) relationship.

There is an opportunity for independent replication of their work with the use of data from Study II of the Ray paper (5) containing a "belief in luck" scale derived from and shown to measure the core concept of the Rotter Locus of Control (LOC) scale (6). The Ss in this study were therefore divided into those above and below the mean on belief in luck, and all relationships were reexamined. There were 55 "internals." They were categorized into those who expected to get 0, 1, or 2 rings on the peg in the Litwin (7) experiment; those who expected to get on 3 or 4 rings; and those who expected to get on 5 or 6 rings. This gave low-, intermediate-, and high-level aspiration groups (ns 26, 17, and 12). All Ss received personality inventories measuring achievement orientation, task orientation, success orientation, fear of failure, and fear of success. The means of the three groups on all inventories were compared, and the Fs were all found not to be significant at the <.05 level. The Wolk and Du Cette results in respect of "internals" were not confirmed.

Some reasons for the nonconfirmation may be as follows: Rather than conducting an experiment in which preferred probability of success actually chosen could be ascertained, Wolk and Du Cette described an imaginary ex periment and asked Ss what probability they would prefer. We may, in other words, be dealing with yet another instance of the attitude-behaviour discrepancy. Further, they did not directly compare motivation scores of people with different levels of aspiration but rather created for each S a "degree of intermediateness" score on level of aspiration. This artificial procedure equates very different levels of aspiration (i.e., very low and very high ones). Their scale of achievement motivation contains at least two items that equate achievement motivation with preference for intermediate risk. The dependent and independent variables were thus artifactually related.

Also contrary to the considerations set out by Wolk and Du Cette, LOC itself in the present study showed no relationship with level of aspiration. They see "internality" and ambition as both leading to intermediate risk preference. In fact, neither did.

Achievement Motivation—Techniques of Developing Achievement Motivation

Motivation can be defined as the driving force behind all the actions of an individual. The influence of an individual's needs and desires both have a strong impact on the direction of their behaviour. Motivation is based on your emotions and achievement-related goals. There are different forms of motivation including extrinsic, intrinsic, physiological, and achievement motivation. There are also more negative forms of motivation. Achievement motivation can be defined as the need for success or the attainment of excellence. Individuals will satisfy their needs through different means, and are driven to succeed for varying reasons both internal and external.

Motivation is the basic drive for all of our actions. Motivation refers to the dynamics of our behaviour, which involves our needs, desires, and ambitions in life. Achievement motivation is based on reaching success and achieving all of our aspirations in life. Achievement goals can affect the way a person performs a task and represent a desire to show competence (Harackiewicz, Barron, Carter, Lehto, & Elliot, 1997). These basic physiological motivational drives affect our natural behaviour in different environments. Most of our goals are incentive-based and can vary from basic hunger to the need for love and the establishment of mature sexual relationships. Our motives for achievement can range from biological needs to satisfying creative desires or realizing success in competitive ventures. Motivation is important because it affects our lives everyday. All of our behaviours, actions, thoughts, and beliefs are influenced by our inner drive to succeed.

Implicit and Self-Attributed Motives

Motivational researchers share the view that achievement behaviour is an interaction between situational variables and the individual subject's motivation to achieve. Two motives are directly involved in the prediction of behaviour, implicit and explicit. Implicit motives are spontaneous impulses to act, also known as task performances, and are aroused through incentives inherent to the task. Explicit motives are expressed through deliberate choices and more often stimulated for extrinsic reasons. Also, individuals with strong implicit needs to achieve goals set higher internal standards, whereas others tend to adhere to the societal norms. These two motives often work together to determine the behaviour of the individual in direction and passion (Brunstein & Maier, 2005).

Explicit and implicit motivations have a compelling impact on behaviour. Task behaviours are accelerated in the face of a challenge through implicit motivation, making performing a task in the most effective manner the primary goal. A person with a strong implicit drive will feel pleasure from achieving a goal in the most efficient way. The increase in effort and overcoming the challenge by mastering the task satisfies the individual. However, the explicit motives are built around a person's self-image. This type of motivation shapes a person's behaviour based on their own self-view and can influence their choices and responses from outside cues. The primary agent for this type of motivation is perception or perceived ability. Many theorists still can not agree whether achievement is based on mastering one's skills or striving to promote a better self-image (Brunstein & Maier, 2005). Most research is still unable to determine whether these different types of motivation would result in different behaviours in the same environment.

The Hierarchal Model of Achievement Motivation

Achievement motivation has been conceptualized in many different ways. Our understanding of achievement-relevant effects, cognition, and behaviour has improved. Despite being similar in nature, many achievement motivation approaches have been developed separately, suggesting that most achievement motivation theories are in concordance with one another instead of competing. Motivational researchers have sought to promote a hierarchal model of approach and avoidance achievement motivation by incorporating the two prominent theories: the achievement motive approach and the achievement goal approach. Achievement motives include the need for achievement and the fear of failure. These are the more predominant motives that direct our behaviour toward positive and negative outcomes. Achievement goals are viewed as more solid cognitive representations pointing individuals toward a specific end. There are three types of these achievement goals: a performance-approach goal, a performance-avoidance goal, and a mastery goal. A performance-approach goal is focused on attaining competence relative to others, a performance-avoidance goal is focused on avoiding incompetence relative to others, and a mastery goal is focused on the development of competence itself and of task mastery. Achievement motives can be seen as direct predictors of achievement-relevant circumstances. Thus, achievement motives are said to have an indirect or distal influence, and achievement goals are said to have a direct or proximal influence on achievement-relevant outcomes (Elliot & McGregor, 1999).

These motives and goals are viewed as working together to regulate achievement behaviour. The hierarchal model presents achievement goals as predictors for performance outcomes. The model is being further conceptualized to include more approaches to achievement motivation. One weakness of the model is that it does not provide an account of the processes responsible for the link between achievement goals and performance. As this model is enhanced, it becomes more useful in predicting the outcomes of achievement-based behaviours (Elliot & McGregor, 1999).

Intrinsic Motivation and Achievement Goals

Intrinsic motivation is defined as the enjoyment of and interest in an activity for its own sake. Fundamentally viewed as an approach form of motivation, intrinsic motivation is identified as an important component of achievement goal theory. Most achievement goal and intrinsic motivational theorists argue that mastery goals are facilitative of intrinsic motivation and related mental processes and performance goals create negative effects. Mastery goals are said to promote intrinsic motivation by fostering perceptions of challenge, encouraging task involvement, generating excitement, and supporting self-determination while performance goals are the opposite. Performance goals are portrayed as undermining intrinsic motivation by instilling perceptions of threat, disrupting task involvement, and creating anxiety and pressure (Elliot & Harackiewicz, 1996).

An alternative set of predictions may be derived from the approach-avoidance framework. Both performance-approach and mastery goals are focused on attaining competence and foster intrinsic motivation. More specifically, in performance-approach or mastery orientations, individuals perceive the achievement setting as a challenge, and this likely will create excitement, encourage cognitive functioning, increase concentration and task absorption, and direct the person toward success and mastery of information which facilitates intrinsic motivation. The performance-avoidance goal is focused on avoiding incompetence, where individuals see the achievement setting as a threat and seek to escape it (Elliot & Harackiewicz, 1996). This orientation is likely to elicit anxiety and withdrawal of effort and cognitive resources while disrupting concentration and motivation.

A Tripartite Model of Motivation for Achievement: Attitude/Drive/Strategy

Motivating students to achieve in school is a topic of great practical concern to teachers and parents, and of great theoretical concern to researchers. New books on the topic appear with increasing frequency and relevant research is proliferating at a rapid rate. Higher education institutions are beginning to provide assistance to students, especially new ones, in developing so-called study skills and self-regulatory skills such as time management. One of the greatest *challenges and opportunities of the 21st century* will be for schools at all levels to focus more on assisting students to become motivated in order that they can succeed in school.

The purpose of this paper is to present a proposed model of motivation for achievement, as applied particularly to the educational setting. This model focuses on three generic variables: (1) *attitude* or beliefs that people hold about themselves, their capabilities, and the factors that account for their outcomes; (2) *drive* or the desire to attain an outcome based on the value people place on it; (3) *strategy* or the techniques that people employ to gain the outcomes they desire. Each of these variables will be described in more detail, and evidence will be provided to support the contention that each exerts an important influence on motivation to achieve in an academic environment.

Achievement outcomes have been regarded as a function of two characteristics, "skill" and "will" (McCombs and Marzano, 1990), and these must be considered separately because possessing the will alone may not insure success if the skill is lacking. The focus in this model is on will, or the motivation to achieve the outcome, and it will be considered separately from level of skill. Where achievement measures such as scores on course examinations or grades are used as criteria of motivation to achieve, measures of skill have to be separated out or controlled for. To measure motivation for achievement directly, measures of *engagement* must be examined.

Cognitive engagement represents the amount of effort spent in either studying or completing assignments. It is the result of motivation, not its source. Pintrich and Schrauben (1992) review a large body of research that suggests that (1) the value of an outcome to the student affects that student's motivation, and (2) motivation leads to cognitive engagement, such engagement manifesting itself in the use or application of various learning strategies.

Many of the studies Pintrich and Schrauben describe employed self-reports of learning strategy use as a measure of cognitive engagement. Such studies become dependent on what students claimed to be doing as a way of determining that they were indeed engaged in a task. To avoid this dependence on students' self-reports, the studies I carried out (either alone or in collaboration with Tom Sexton) and report on in this paper operationalized cognitive engagement as a manifestation of effort expenditure or actual performance on the homework task of writing test items on text chapters in which students had the option to perform assignments for extra credit. In studies I carried out and report on using achievement test scores as a measure of motivation to achieve, relevant data on students' skill level was used as a control.

Motivation in Classroom Context

Power in the Classroom

Prior to presenting some of these motivational strategies, it would be of relevance to say a few things about the teacher/ learner relationship. Whichever way we look at it, this relationship is riddled with power and status. For many, power plays a large part in the relationship. The rights and duties of teachers and learners are related to power. For example, many teachers might assert that they have the right to punish those learners who misbehave. In any social encounter involving two or more people, there are certain power relationships 'which are almost always asymmetrical' (Wright, 1987: 17). Social psychologists distinguish between three different types of power—*coercive*, *reward-based*, and *referent* (ibid.). The basis of coercive power is punishment. Some individuals or institutions have the authority to punish others. The basis of the second type of power is reward. Some individuals or institutions have the power to reward what they deem appropriate behaviour. For example, business organisations reward employees with a salary, a bonus etc. The basis of the third type of power is motivation. In this case, individuals or institutions appeal to the commitment and interest of others. In view of this three-fold paradigm, it is of importance to concern ourselves with the fostering of learner motivation, as it is considered to be the most effective and proactive, so to speak, power relationship.

Group Processes and Motivation

A discussion of motivation and motivational strategies would not be complete without a consideration of group processes, inasmuch as there is usually a group of people that we as teachers are called on to motivate. Tuckman (1969, quoted in Argyle, 1969) established that a group went through four stages from its formation, which has important implications for the study of the classroom and the use of group activities during teaching.

- Stage 1 ***Forming***: At first, there is some anxiety among the members of the group, as they are dependent on the leader (that is, the teacher) and they have to find out what behaviour is acceptable.
- Stage 2 ***Storming***: There is conflict between sub-groups and rebellion against the leader. Members of the group resist their leader and the role relations attending the function of the group are questioned.
- Stage 3 ***Norming***: The group begins to develop a sort of cohesion. Members of the group begin to support each other. At this stage, there is co-operation and open exchange of views and feelings about their roles and each other.

- Stage 4 ***Performing***: Most problems are resolved and there is a great deal of interpersonal activity. Everyone is devoted to completing the tasks they have been assigned.

Experience shows that almost every group goes through these four (or even more) stages until it reaches equilibrium and, thus, taps into its potential. In reality, this process may go on forever, since student lethargy and underachievement norms in the classroom are considered to be basic hindrances to effective teaching and learning (Daniels, 1994). Against this background, we will try to design a framework for motivational strategies.

Competition and Co-operation

When it comes to interaction and group dynamics, there are two particular factors that can hinder or facilitate group achievement: competition of Co-operation (Deutsch, 2003). Within a group or team setting, the two factors of Co-operation and competition can either propel the team to success or consign the group's effort to failure depending on which factor is dominant. Co-operation is "work[ing] or act[ing] together or jointly for a common purpose or benefit (cooperate). Competition, on the other hand, takes place when people "strive to gain or win something by defeating or establishing superiority over others who are trying to do the same thing" (Oxford American Dictionaries).

Deutsch suggests six "cooperative relations" in which he describes six positive characteristics that make Co-operation within a group more likely. These six factors include: 1. Effective communication. 2. Friendliness, helpfulness, and less obstructiveness. 3. Coordination of effort, divisions of labour, orientation of task achievements, orderliness in discussion, and high productivity. 4. Feelings of agreement with the ideas of others and a sense of basic similarity in beliefs in one's own ideas and in the value that other members attach to those ideas. 5. The willingness to enhance the other's power (as others capabilities are strengthened, you are strengthened). 6. Defining conflicting interests as a mutual problem to be solved by collaborative effort (Deustch). In his six points, Deustch articulates the ideal features one would expect to find in an environment of a cooperative organization. And just as these factors contribute toward the cooperativeness of a group, one would find the opposite characteristics prevalent in a group where internal or in-group competition prevails. Poor communication, obstructiveness and lack of helpfulness (Deustch, 2003), and group disorder, disagreement and the critical rejection of ideas (Deustch), and striving to "enhance one's own power" (Deutsch,2003) sum up the "conflicting relations."

An example of Co-operation versus competition can be found in a study called The Prisoner's Dilemma (Dixit and Nalebuff). In this tradeoff, two criminals (we'll call them 1 and 2) are arrested on the "suspicion of having committed armed robbery and sure enough they are found to be carrying concealed weapons" (Dixit and Nalebuff). The police are able to talk to the suspects separately and both are given an opportunity to confess or "rat out" the other person. In this situation, there are four plausible and equally likely outcomes. In the first, both parties could cooperate with each other and refuse to confess or turn his or her partner in. The outcome of this condition is most beneficial for both individuals in that they are most like to receive a light sentence as a result of being armed, but not a long sentence for the actual crime. In the second and third situations, one of the individuals "rats out" the other and therefore he receives a light sentence while his partner receives a longer sentence for the crime. In this state of affairs, there is a sort of competition where there are conflicting interests amongst the two individuals. In the final circumstance both individuals rat each other out, are convicted and found guilty, and both serve equally long sentences in prison.

Leadership Traits

One of the most important contributions psychology has made to the field of business has been in determining the key traits of acknowledged leaders. Psychological tests have been used to determine what characteristics are most commonly noted among successful leaders. This list of characteristics can be used for developmental purposes to help managers gain insight and develop their leadership skills. The increasing rate of change in the business environment is a major factor in this emphasis on leadership. Whereas in the past, managers were expected to maintain the status quo in order to move ahead, new forces in the marketplace have made it necessary to expand this narrow focus. The new leaders of tomorrow are visionary. They are both learners and teachers. Not only do they foresee paradigm changes in society, but they also have a strong sense of ethics and work to build integrity in their organizations. Raymond Cattell, a pioneer in the field of personality assessment, developed the Leadership Potential equation in 1954. This equation, which was based on a study of military leaders, is used today to determine the traits which characterize an effective leader. The traits of an effective leader include the following:

- Emotional stability. Good leaders must be able to tolerate frustration and stress. Overall, they must be well-adjusted and have the psychological maturity to deal with anything they are required to face.
- Dominance. Leaders are often times competitive and decisive and usually enjoy overcoming obstacles. Overall, they are assertive in their thinking style as well as their attitude in dealing with others.
- Enthusiasm. Leaders are usually seen as active, expressive, and energetic. They are often very optimistic and open to change. Overall, they are generally quick and alert and tend to be uninhibited.
- Conscientiousness. Leaders are often dominated by a sense of duty and tend to be very exacting in character. They usually have a very high standard of excellence and an inward desire to do one's best. They also have a need for order and tend to be very self-disciplined.
- Social boldness. Leaders tend to be spontaneous risk-takers. They are usually socially aggressive and generally thick-skinned. Overall, they are responsive to others and tend to be high in emotional stamina.

- Tough-mindedness. Good leaders are practical, logical, and to-the-point. They tend to be low in sentimental attachments and comfortable with criticism. They are usually insensitive to hardship and overall, are very poised.
- Self-assurance. Self-confidence and resiliency are common traits among leaders. They tend to be free of guilt and have little or no need for approval. They are generally secure and free from guilt and are usually unaffected by prior mistakes or failures.
- Compulsiveness. Leaders were found to be controlled and very precise in their social interactions. Overall, they were very protective of their integrity and reputation and consequently tended to be socially aware and careful, abundant in foresight, and very careful when making decisions or determining specific actions.

Beyond these basic traits, leaders of today must also possess traits which will help them motivate others and lead them in new directions. Leaders of the future must be able to envision the future and convince others that their vision is worth following. To do this, they must have the following personality traits:

- High energy. Long hours and some travel are usually a prerequisite for leadership positions, especially as your company grows. Remaining alert and staying focused are two of the greatest obstacles you will have to face as a leader.
- Intuitiveness. Rapid changes in the world today combined with information overload result in an inability to "know" everything. In other words, reasoning and logic will not get you through all situations. In fact, more and more leaders are learning to the value of using their intuition and trusting their own instincts when making decisions.
- Maturity. To be a good leader, personal power and recognition must be secondary to the development of your employees. In other words, maturity is based on recognizing that more can be accomplished by empowering others than can be by ruling others.

- Team orientation. Business leaders today put a strong emphasis on team work. Instead of promoting an adult/child relationship with their employees, leaders create an adult/adult relationship which fosters team cohesiveness.
- Empathy. Being able to put yourself in the other person's shoes is a key trait of leaders. Without empathy, you can't build trust. And without trust, you will never be able to get the best effort from your employees.
- Charisma. People usually perceive leaders as larger than life. Charisma plays a large part in this perception. Leaders who have charisma are able to arouse strong emotions in their employees by defining a vision which unites and captivates them. Using this vision, leaders motivate employees to reach toward a future goal by tying the goal to substantial personal rewards and values. Personal traits play a major role in determining who will and who will not be comfortable leading others.

However, it is important to remember that people are forever learning and changing. Leaders are rarely (if ever) born. Circumstances and persistence are major components in the developmental process of any leader. If your goal is to become a leader, work on developing those areas from the list above that you are weak in. For instance, if you have all of the basic traits, but do not consider yourself very much of a people person, take classes or read books on empathy. Get feedback from others on how they see you and what they think you can do to develop those traits. There are many leadership training programs around. Contact your local business school to find one near you.

Leadership Styles

The study of leadership styles take into consideration what a leader does, says, and how he acts. It has to do with the study of the leader's approach to the use of authority and the resultant participation of others in decision-making. A closer examination of some selected leadership styles reveal the magnitude of the leader's responsibility those with whom he works. Lall and

Lall (1979) listed these five styles of leadership with their definitions as follows:

Autocratic Leadership

The autocratic leader gets vested authority through the office more than from personal attributes. He seeks little group participation in decision-making.

Advantage: The leader generally gets things done.

Disadvantage: The follower becomes dependent on the leader and his personal development is jeopardized.

Bureaucratic Leadership

This style f leadership is based on the utilization of a system of files to solve problems. It can be styled as leadership by centralization.

Advantage: There is a ready system on hand to embark upon the solution of problems.

Disadvantage: It is too well organized and tends to depersonalize the organization.

Charismatic Leadership

Here the leader focuses attention on himself. He appears to possess a certain charisma and followers are converted to and are champions of the cause.

Advantage: The leader gets a lot of individuals to accept his views and defend his cause.

Disadvantage: These leaders tend to lean towards authoritarian or bureaucratic styles of leadership.

Laissez-Faire Leadership

Complete permissiveness is allowed in this style of leadership. The group lacks direction because the leader does not help in making-decision.

Advantage: Every follower has the opportunity to make decisions.

Disadvantage: This style can easily lead to anarchy if allowed to function for a long period of time.

Democratic Leadership

In this style of leadership most policies derive from group decision. The leader is involved in policy formation but does not dominate group action.

Advantage: Individual growth is enhancing through participation in the organization's operations.

Disadvantage: The possibility of the sidelining of leadership initiative as a result of majority group decision.

One of the first and most famous studies of leadership style was conducted by Lewin, Lippit, and White (1939) where they placed selected individuals into various groups with different leadership styles. The styles chosen were democratic, in which group decisions were made by majority vote, equal participation was encouraged and criticism and punishment were minimal; autocratic, in which all decisions were made by the leader and participants were required to follow prescribed procedures under strict discipline; and laissez-faire, in which the actual leadership activity of the group leader was kept at a minimum, allowing the participants to work and play essentially without supervision.

The groups with democratic style of leadership were the most satisfied and functional in the most orderly and positive manner. The number and degree of aggressive acts were greatest in the autocratically led groups.

From the review of leadership theories, it is obvious that there is no one best leadership style. Hein and Nicholson (1968) argue that leaders are rarely totally people—or task-oriented; leader, followers, situation all influence leadership effectiveness and therefore an integrating of leadership theories seems appropriate. This type of approach reflects an escapist mentality that will settle for anything as long as he gets out of the present dilemma.

Is there a more excellent style of leadership? There must be another style of leadership that can provide for the upward mobility of followers void of the superordinate-subordinate syndrome; facilitatory leadership with vision. In my own search for a leadership style that makes a difference, I have discovered another model, which has broadened my vision of ministry: servanthood.

Classroom Climate

In all classroom settings with which the writer is familiar, the teacher is the designated leader and the students are the followers. A set of rules and regulations, as well as designated punishments for breaking those rules, is placed in a highly visible position in front of the students. It has generally been assumed that formal structures permit the leaders to function effectively, help members perform their tasks, and see that the purpose of the group has been achieved (Bany & Johnson, 1964). In classes where rule infractions are overly stressed, and the pupils criticized, the writer has observed a large amount of reporting and blaming others, on the part of the students. The children also seem unable to work together collaboratively.

In classes where the need for rules is discussed with the children, and the children are encouraged to understand why rules are needed and how they can help each other follow the rules, there is a minimum of scapegoating and tale-telling.

In order to be able to follow rules, children have to develop a sense of responsibility. This is a maturational task that includes emotional, social, and psychological growth.

Unit-VIII

Personality and Assessment

Meaning and Definitions of Personality

Main the measurement of personal characteristics. Assessment is an end result of gathering information intended to advance psychological theory and research and to increase the probability that wise decisions will be made in applied settings (e.g., in selecting the most promising people from a group of job applicants). The approach taken by the specialist in personality assessment is based on the assumption that much of the observable variability in behaviour from one person to another results from differences in the extent to which individuals possess particular underlying personal characteristics (traits). The assessment specialist seeks to define these traits, to measure them objectively, and to relate them to socially significant aspects of behaviour.

A distinctive feature of the scientific approach to personality measurement is the effort, wherever possible, to describe human characteristics in quantitative terms. How much of a trait manifests itself in an individual? How many traits are present? Quantitative personality measurement is especially useful in comparing groups of people as well as individuals. Do groups of people from different cultural and economic backgrounds differ when considered in the light of their particular personality attributes or traits? How large are the group differences?

Overt behaviour is a reflection of interactions among a wide range of underlying factors, including the bodily state of the individual and the effects of that person's past personal experiences. Hence, a narrowly focused approach is inadequate to do justice to the complex human behaviour that occurs under the constantly changing set of challenges, pleasures, demands, and stresses of everyday life. The sophisticated measurement of human personality inescapably depends on the use of a variety of concepts to provide trait definitions and entails the application of various methods of observation and evaluation. Personality theorists and researchers seek to define and to understand the diversity of human traits, the many ways people have of thinking and perceiving and learning and emoting. Such nonmaterial human dimensions, types, and attributes are constructs—in this case, inferences drawn from observed behaviour. Widely studied personality constructs include anxiety, hostility, emotionality, motivation, and introversion-extroversion. Anxiety, for example, is a concept, or construct, inferred in people from what they say, their facial expressions, and their body movements.

Personality is interactional in two senses. As indicated above, personal characteristics can be thought of as products of interactions among underlying psychological factors; for example, an individual may experience tension because he or she is both shy and desirous of social success. These products, in turn, interact with the types of situations people confront in their daily lives. A person who is anxious about being evaluated might show debilitated performance in evaluative situations (for example, taking tests), but function well in other situations in which an evaluative emphasis is not present. Personality makeup can be either an asset or a liability depending on the situation. For example, some people approach evaluative situations with fear and foreboding, while others seem to be motivated in a desirable direction by competitive pressures associated with performance.

Personality is the supreme realization of the innate idiosyncrasy of a living being. It is an act of high courage flung in the face of life, the absolute affirmation of all that constitutes the individual, the most successful adaptation to the universal condition of existence coupled with the greatest possible freedom for self-determination."-Carl Gustav Jung, 1934.

As we move from Intelligence to Personality

As this course moves from intelligence (1st 5 weeks) into personality (next 10 weeks), it is worth pointing out that the relationship between intelligence and personality may be stronger than many assume.

Intelligence influences different aspects of personality in many different ways. In fact, intelligence is sometimes considered to be part of personality. This issue will probably always be debated. The main point to bear in mind is that both intelligence and personality are prominent individual differences.

Personality is not easily defined. Basically, 'personality' refers to our attempts to capture or summarize an individual's 'essence'. Personality is personality, the science of describing and understanding persons. Clearly, personality is a core area of study for psychology, if not the core. Together with intelligence, the topic of personality constitutes the most significant area of individual difference study.

No two people are exactly the same-not even identical twins. Some people are anxious, some are risk-taking; some are phlegmatic, some highly-strung; some are confident, some shy; and some are quiet and some are loquacious. This issue of differences is fundamental to the study of personality. Note also that in studying these differences we will also examine where the differences come from: as with intelligence we will find that there is a mixture of nature and nurture involved.

Perspectives on personality that we'll be examining:

- Trait Perspective
- Biological Perspective
- Psychoanalytic Perspective
- Learning Perspective
- Phenomenological Perspective
- Cognitive Perspective

Various Definitions of Personality

- "Deceptive masquerade or mimicry."

- "The entire organization of a human being at any stage of development."
- "Levels or layers of dispositions, usually with a unifying or integrative principle at the top."
- "The integration of those systems or habits that represent an individual's characteristic adjustments to the environment."
- "The way in which the person does such things as remembering, thinking or loving."
- "Those characteristics that account for consistent patterns of behaviour"
- "Personality is not an existing substantive entity to be searched for but a complex construct to be developed and defined by the observer." (Smith & Vetter, 1982, p.5)
- A contemporary definition for personality is offered by Carver and Scheier (2000, p.5): "Personality is a dynamic organisation, inside the person, of psychophysical systems that create a person's characteristic patterns of behaviour, thoughts, and feelings." Carver & Scheier (2000, p.5)
    - o Dynamic Organisation: suggests ongoing readjustments, adaptation to experience, continual upgrading and maintaining Personality doesn't just lie there. It has process and it's organised.
    - o Inside the Person: suggests internal storage of patterns, supporting the notion that personality influences behaviours, etc.
    - o Psychophysical systems: suggests that the physical is also involved in 'who we are'

      Characteristic Patterns: implies that consistency/ continuity which are uniquely identifying of an individual
    - o Behaviour, Thoughts, and Feelings: indicates that personality includes a wide range of psychological experience/manifestation: that personality is displayed in MANY ways.

- Carver & Scheier (2000, p.5) suggest that the word personality "conveys a sense of consistency, internal causality, and personal distinctiveness". This issue of "personal distinctiveness is very important. There are certain universal characteristics of the human race and particular features of individuals. We all for example experience stress and the elevated cortisol that goes with it, and we all suffer the immune suppressive effects thereof. BUT each of us is unique too.

Major Determinants of Personality

Personality is the outcome of a continuous personal quality development process. The role of personality becomes clear in a particular situation. Personality is recognised in a situation. It is the result of personal quality interaction in a particular condition. The major determinants of personality of an individual are given below:

Biological Factors

Heredity: Heredity refers to those factors that were determined at conception. Physical stature, facial attractiveness, sex, temperament, muscle composition and reflexes, energy level, and biological rhythms are characteristics that are generally considered to be either completely or substantially influenced by who your parents were; that is, by their biological, physiological, and inherent psychological makeup. The contribution of heredity to personality development is vividly clear for developing external appearance, behaviour, social stimuli, self inner awareness, organising traits, etc.

Brain: Brain has a great impact on personality. The psychologists are unable to prove empirically the contribution of human brain in influencing personality. Father and children generally adopt the same type of brain stimulation. The differences are caused by environment. Electrical stimulation of brain (ESB) and split brain psychology (SBP) are the outcome of genetic transmission. The are helpful in moulding employee's behaviour. ESB is used for motivating employees towards better performances. Managers are trained to use SBP for mobilising employees for proper behaviour.

Physical Features: Perhaps the most outstanding factor that contributes to personality is the physical stature of an individual. An individual's external appearance is proved to be having a tremendous effect on personality. For example, the fact that a person is short or tall, fat or thin, handsome or ugly, black or whitish will undoubtedly influence the person's effect on others and in turn will affect the self-concept. A person's physical characteristics may be related to his approach to the social environment, to the expectancies of others, and to their reactions, to him. These in turn may have impact on personality development.

Theories of Personality—Type, Trait, Type and Trait, Psychoanalytic

Critics of personality theory claim personality is "plastic" across time, places, moods, and situations. Changes in personality may indeed result from diet (or lack thereof), medical effects, significant events, or learning. However, most personality theories emphasize stability over fluctuation.

Trait Theories

According to the *Diagnostic and Statistical Manual* of the American Psychiatric Association, personality traits are "enduring patterns of perceiving, relating to, and thinking about the environment and oneself that are exhibited in a wide range of social and personal contexts." Theorists generally assume a) traits are relatively stable over time, b) traits differ among individuals (e.g. some people are outgoing while others are reserved), and c) traits influence behaviour.

The most common models of traits incorporate three to five broad dimensions or factors. The least controversial dimension, observed as far back as the ancient Greeks, is simply extraversion vs. introversion (outgoing and physical-stimulation-oriented vs. quiet and physical-stimulation-averse).

- **Gordon Allport** delineated different kinds of traits, which he also called dispositions. *Central traits* are basic to an individual's personality, while *secondary traits* are more peripheral. *Common traits* are those recognized within a culture and thus may vary from culture to culture. *Cardinal traits* are those by which an individual may be strongly recognized.

- **Raymond Cattell's** research propagated a two-tiered personality structure with sixteen "primary factors" (16 Personality Factors) and five "secondary factors."
- **Hans Eysenck**, who believed just three traits-extraversion, neuroticism and psychoticism-were sufficient to describe human personality. Differences between Cattell and Eysenck emerged due to preferences for different forms of factor analysis, with Cattell using oblique, Eysenck orthogonal, rotation to analyse the factors that emerged when personality questionnaires were subjected to statistical analysis. Today, the Big Five factors have the weight of a considerable amount of empirical research behind them. Building on the work of Cattell and others.
- **Lewis Goldberg** proposed a five-dimension personality model, nicknamed the "Big Five":
  1. Extraversion-outgoing and stimulation-oriented vs. quiet and stimulation-avoiding
  2. Neuroticism-emotionally reactive, prone to negative emotions vs. calm, imperturbable, optimistic
  3. Agreeableness-affable, friendly, conciliatory vs. aggressive, dominant, disagreeable
  4. Conscientiousness-dutiful, planful, and orderly vs. laidback, spontaneous, and unreliable
  5. Openness to experience-open to new ideas and change vs. traditional and oriented toward routine

  For ease of remembrance, this can be written as either OCEAN or CANOE.
- **John L. Holland's** *RIASEC* vocational model, commonly referred to as the **Holland Codes**, stipulates there are six personality traits that lead people to choose their career paths. This model is widely used in vocational counselling and is a circumplex model where the six types are represented as a hexagon where

adjacent types are more closely related than those more distant.

Trait models have been criticized as being purely descriptive and offering little explanation of the underlying causes of personality. Eysenck's theory, however, does propose biological mechanisms as driving traits, and modern behaviour genetics researchers have demonstrated a clear genetic substrate to them. Another potential weakness with trait theories is they lead people to accept oversimplified classifications, or worse offer advice, based on a superficial analysis of one's personality. Finally, trait models often underestimate the effect of specific situations on people's behaviour. It is important to remember traits are statistical generalizations that do not always correspond to an individual's behaviour.

Type Theories

Personality type refers to the psychological classification of different types of people. Personality types are distinguished from personality traits, which come in different levels or degrees. According to type theories, for example, there are two types of people, introverts and extraverts. According to trait theories, introversion and extraversion are part of a continuous dimension, with many people in the middle. The idea of psychological types originated in the theoretical work of Carl Jung and William Marston, whose work is reviewed in Dr. Travis Bradberry's *The Personality Code*. Jung's seminal 1921 book on the subject is available in English as *Psychological Types*.

Building on the writings and observations of Carl Jung, during World War II, Isabel Briggs Myers and her mother, Katharine C. Briggs, delineated personality types by constructing the Myers-Briggs Type Indicator. This model was later used by David Keirsey with a different understanding from Jung, Briggs and Myers. In the former Soviet Union, Lithuanian Auora Augustinavieiute independently derived a model of personality type from Jung's called Socionics.

The model is an older and more theoretical approach to personality, accepting extraversion and introversion as basic psychological orientations in connection with two pairs of psychological functions:

- Perceiving functions: sensing and intuition (trust in concrete, sensory-oriented facts vs. trust in abstract concepts and imagined possibilities)
- Judging functions: thinking and feeling (basing decisions primarily on logic vs. considering the effect on people).

Briggs and Myers also added another personality dimension to their type indicator to measure whether a person prefers to use a judging or perceiving function when interacting with the external world. Therefore they included questions designed to indicate whether someone wishes to come to conclusions (judgment) or to keep options open (perception).

This personality typology has some aspects of a trait theory: it explains people's behaviour in terms of opposite fixed characteristics. In these more traditional models, the sensing/intuition preference is considered the most basic, dividing people into "N" (intuitive) or "S" (sensing) personality types. An "N" is further assumed to be guided either by thinking or feeling, and divided into the "NT" (scientist, engineer) or "NF" (author, humanitarian) temperament. An "S", by contrast, is assumed to be guided more by the judgment/perception axis, and thus divided into the "SJ" (guardian, traditionalist) or "SP" (performer, artisan) temperament.

These four are considered basic, with the other two factors in each case (including always extraversion/introversion) less important. Critics of this traditional view have observed that the types can be quite strongly stereotyped by professions (although neither Myers nor Keirsey engaged in such stereotyping in their type descriptions), and thus may arise more from the need to categorize people for purposes of guiding their career choice. This among other objections led to the emergence of the five factor view, which is less concerned with behaviour under work conditions and more concerned with behaviour in personal and emotional circumstances. Some critics have argued for more or fewer dimensions while others have proposed entirely different theories (often assuming different definitions of "personality").

Type A personality: During the 1950s, Meyer Friedman and his co-workers defined what they called Type A and Type B behaviour patterns. They theorized that intense, hard-driving Type A personalities had a higher risk of coronary disease because they are "stress junkies." Type B people, on the other hand, tended to be relaxed, less competitive, and lower in risk. There was also a Type AB mixed profile. Dr. Redford Williams, cardiologist at Duke University, refuted Friedman's theory that Type A personalities have a higher risk of coronary heart disease; however, current research indicates that only the hostility component of Type A may have health implications. Type A/B theory has been extensively criticized by psychologists because it tends to oversimplify the many dimensions of an individual's personality.

Psychoanalytic Theories

Psychoanalytic theories explain human behaviour in terms of the interaction of various components of personality. Sigmund Freud was the founder of this school. Freud drew on the physics of his day (thermodynamics) to coin the term psychodynamics. Based on the idea of converting heat into mechanical energy, he proposed psychic energy could be converted into behaviour. Freud's theory places central importance on dynamic, unconscious psychological conflicts. Freud divides human personality into three significant components: the ego, superego, and id. The **id** acts according to the *pleasure principle*, demanding immediate gratification of its needs regardless of external environment; the **ego** then must emerge in order to realistically meet the wishes and demands of the id in accordance with the outside world, adhering to the *reality principle*. Finally, the **superego** inculcates moral judgment and societal rules upon the ego, thus forcing the demands of the id to be met not only realistically but morally. The superego is the last function of the personality to develop, and is the embodiment of parental/social ideals established during childhood. According to Freud, personality is based on the dynamic interactions of these three components.

The channeling and release of sexual (libidal) and aggressive energies, which ensues from the "Eros" (sex; instinctual self-preservation) and "Thanatos" (death; instinctual self-annihilation) drives respectively, are major components of his theory. It is important to note Freud's broad understanding of sexuality included all kinds of pleasurable feelings experienced by the human body.

Freud proposed five psychosexual stages of personality development. He believed adult personality is dependent upon early childhood experiences and largely determined by age five. Fixations that develop during the Infantile stage contribute to adult personality and behaviour.

One of Sigmund Freud's earlier associates, Alfred Adler, did agree with Freud early childhood experiences are important to development, and believed birth order may influence personality development. Adler believed the oldest was the one that set high goals to achieve to get the attention they lost back when the younger siblings were born. He believed the middle children were competitive and ambitious possibly so they are able to surpass the first-born's achievements, but were not as much concerned about the glory. Also he believed the last born would be more dependent and sociable but be the baby. He also believed that the only child loves being the centre of attention and matures quickly, but in the end fails to become independent.

Heinz Kohut thought similarly to Freud's idea of transference. He used narcissism as a model of how we develop our sense of self. Narcissism is the exaggerated sense of one self in which is believed to exist in order to protect one's low self esteem and sense of worthlessness. Kohut had a significant impact on the field by extending Freud's theory of narcissism and introducing what he called the 'self-object transferences' of mirroring and idealization. In other words, children need to idealize and emotionally "sink into" and identify with the idealized competence of admired figures such as parents or older siblings. They also need to have their self-worth mirrored by these people. These experiences allow them to thereby learn the self-soothing and other skills that are necessary for the development of a healthy sense of self.

Another important figure in the world of personality theory was Karen Horney. She is credited with the development of the "real self" and the "ideal self". She believes all people have these two views of their own self. The "real self" is how you really are with regards to personality, values, and morals; but the "ideal self" is a construct you apply to yourself to conform to social and personal norms and goals. Ideal self would be "I can be successful, I am CEO material"; and real self would be "I just work in the mail room, with not much chance of high promotion".

Assessment of Personality: Projective and Non-Projective Techniques

One group of assessment specialists believes that the more freedom people have in picking their responses, the more meaningful the description and classification that can be obtained. Because personality inventories do not permit much freedom of choice, some researchers and clinicians prefer to use projective techniques, in which a person is shown ambiguous stimuli (such as shapes or pictures) and asked to interpret them in some way. (Such stimuli allow relative freedom in projecting one's own interests and feelings into them, reacting in any way that seems appropriate.) Projective techniques are believed to be sensitive to unconscious dimensions of personality. Defense mechanisms, latent impulses, and anxieties have all been inferred from data gathered in projective situations.

Personality inventories and projective techniques do have some elements in common; inkblots, for example, are ambiguous, but so also are many of the statements on inventories such as the MMPI. These techniques differ in that the subject is given substantially free rein in responding to projective stimuli rather than merely answering true or false, for example. Another similarity between projective and questionnaire or inventory approaches is that all involve the use of relatively standardized testing situations.

While projective techniques are often lumped together as one general methodology, in actual practice there are several approaches to assessment from a projective point of view. Although projective techniques share the common characteristic that they permit the subject wide latitude in responding, they still may be distinguished broadly as follows: (1) associative techniques, in which the subject is asked to react to words, to inkblots, or to other stimuli with the first associated thoughts that come to mind; (2) construction techniques, in which the subject is asked to create something—for example, make up a story or draw a self-portrait; (3) completion techniques, in which the subject is asked to finish a partially developed stimulus, such as adding the last words to an incomplete sentence; (4) choice or ordering techniques, in which the subject is asked to choose from among or to give some orderly sequence to stimuli—for example, to choose from or arrange a set of pictures or inkblots; (5) expressive techniques, in which the subject is asked to use free expression in some manner, such as in finger painting.

Hidden personality defense mechanisms, latent emotional impulses, and inner anxieties all have been attributed to test takers by making theoretical inferences from data gathered as they responded in projective situations. While projective stimuli are ambiguous, they are usually administered under fairly standardized conditions. Quantitative (numerical) measures can be derived from subjects' responses to them. These include the number of responses one makes to a series of inkblots and the number of responses to the blots in which the subject perceives what seem to him to be moving animals.

Remember that we defined learning as "a relatively permanent change in behaviour (or behaviour potential) as a result of experience or practice." Remember also that we said maturation, or relatively permanent change as a result of biology and genetics, is the only other explanation for relatively permanent change. That is, when a person is different today than he or she was yesterday, or last week, or last month or last year, etc. it is because that person either matured or learned something, or both. When both of these occur simultaneously, in a way that is difficult to study independently, we refer to that as development. In addition, development has the connotation of improvement or increase in complexity or level. In reality, most of what we do in education has both learning (i.e., providing experiences for students) and maturational (appropriate for a given biological functioning) aspects. However, in this course we will focus mainly on learning with less emphasis on development. The major exception is when we study the cognitive theory of Jean Piaget.

Another important issue in the area of teaching and learning is the difference between aptitude and achievement. By aptitude we mean the potential one has to learn and/or develop. Aptitude is a measurement in the present that is intended to predict future events, especially the capacity of an individual to learn (i.e., change as a result of experience or practice.). IQ is a measure of academic aptitude. Students with higher academic aptitude will show more achievement than students with low academic aptitude if both are given the same quality and amount of experience or practice. Other examples include manual dexterity, spatial, mechanical, musical, etc. Achievement, on the other hand, refers to capacities or skills or knowledge one has now that one did not have in the past. That is, achievement is a measurement in the present that refers to behaviour or effort or learning done in the past. It is especially important that our educational system not mix the two. Achievement is likely the result of specific training or experiences whereas aptitude is more likely the result of genetic inheritance and general experiences that may or may not have been explicitly provided to all students. If some students have been provided appropriate learning experiences, while others have not, we should not use achievement measures as measures of aptitude. Rather we need to provide students with specific learning experiences, making sure that they have the prerequisite skills necessary to learn, before we make judgments about aptitude.

Another important distinction is between instruction, assessment, and evaluation. Remember that assessment refers to the collection of data to describe or better understand an issue whereas evaluation refers to the comparison of data to a standard for the purpose of judging worth or quality. Instruction is defined as "the purposeful direction of student learning" and is one of the three major categories of teacher classroom behaviour (the other two are planning and managment.) Instruction, then, is providing experiences for learners that will allow them to successfully move from their present level of knowledge, skill, etc. to a desired level. It is an active process involving both teachers and students moving towards specific desired end results. In relation to instruction, assessment is the collection of data before, during, and after instruction. Evaluation is the process of making judgments at these specified times. When done before instruction we might make decisions as to a student's having the prerequisite skills or the necessary aptitude to learn the material in the specified time allotted. During instruction, we might make decisions about the appropriateness of the student effort or student learning. After instruction, we can make decisions about whether or not the student has mastered the material sufficiently to go on to the next learning experience.

In future presentations we will discuss the concept of "What You Measure Is What You Get" (WYMIWYG) which highlights the tendency to focus during instruction on those outcomes you intend to measure or that will measured by some outside individual or agency. In addition, we will discuss how the changing requirements of the information age demand that educators focus on important outcomes such as critical thinking and social skills in addition to achievement in basic skills such as reading and mathematics.

Another issue already discussed is related to reliability and validity. Both are important for every aspect of evaluation and research. Reliablity refers to the consistency or the dependability of the data whereas validity refers to the truthfulness or correctness of the data. As previously stated, assessment data and evaluation decisions may be reliable (consistent) without being valid (correctly judging the truth of the data relative to intentions.) However, the reverse is not true (i.e., data cannot be valid if they are not reliable.)

Three issues are important for classroom assessment that is under the control of the teacher. The first relates to what data (assessments and measures) we will use for making judgments. The issue of traditional versus performance assessment is important in this regard. By traditional assessment we are referring to the types of assessments generally found in classrooms: multiple-choice, true-false, or matching objective exams or fill-in-the-blank, short-answer, or essay exams. Performance assessment, on the other hand, refers to data collected during the actual accomplishment or demonstration of a particular set of skills or knowledge. A major difference is that traditional assessment is almost always done out of context (i.e., separate and apart from the situation in which it will be used.) Performance assessment, on the other hand, includes as much of the context as possible. It may be that a student fixes an engine, or perhaps gives a speech to a group of parents. In any case, the situation is as real as possible. A second issue, that of formative versus summative assessment, is an issue of timing of assessment and evaluation. Formative assessment refers to any data collection that occurs before or during instruction. If it is done prior to instruction for the purpose of determining a students readiness for instruction, we call that diagnostic assessment. Summative assessment is done at the end of instruction to determine what has been learned. There is no expectation of further instruction at that point.

The third issue is one of the most important issues in measurement and evaluation: the difference between criterion- and norm-referenced testing. In general, criterion-referenced testing is done when we want to know how much a student knows vis-a-vis a pre-set standard and norm-referenced testing is done when we want to know how one student or group of students compares to other students in terms of the content or skills being tested. It's important to be knowledgeable regarding this issues so that you can explain test results to students and parents.

Aptitude—Concept, Types and Measurement

An **aptitude** is an innate, acquired or learned or developed component of a competency (*being the others: knowledge, understanding and attitude*) to do a certain kind of work at a certain level. Aptitudes may be physical or mental. The innate nature of aptitude is in contrast to achievement, which represents knowledge or ability that is gained.

Intelligence and Aptitudes

Aptitude and intelligence quotient are related, and in some ways opposite, views of human mental ability. Whereas intelligence quotient sees intelligence as being a single measurable characteristic affecting all mental ability, aptitude breaks mental ability down into many different characteristics which are supposed to be more or less independent of each other. On the contrary, casual analysis with any group of test scores will nearly always show them to be highly correlated. The U.S. Department of Labour's General Learning Ability, for instance, is determined by combining Verbal, Numerical and Spatial aptitude subtests. In a given person some may be relatively low and others relatively high. In the context of an aptitude test the "high" and "low" scores are usually not far apart, because all ability test scores tend to be correlated. Aptitude is better applied intra-individually to determine what tasks a given individual is relatively more skilled at performing. Inter-individual aptitude differences are typically not very significant due to IQ differences. Of course this assumes individuals have not already been pre-screened for IQ through some other process such as SAT scores, GRE scores, finishing medical school, etc.

Aptitude Only Batteries

Aptitudes are generally tested in the form of an aptitude battery which tests a large number of aptitudes at one time with a series of small tests for each aptitude. Aptitude batteries may lean more toward innate aptitudes or more toward learned skills. Aptitude batteries that lean toward aptitudes are often useful in selecting a career. The leading researchers and purveyors of aptitude tests are:

- The Vocational Research Institute which produces a test used in schools and agencies that combines interest and aptitude for career guidance is Careerscope.
- The Johnson O'Connor Research Foundation (JORF) is the original aptitude assessment organization. It produces the Johnson O'Connor Aptitude Battery (JOAB).

- The Highlands Company is a spin-off of the Johnson O'Connor Research Foundation. It produces and the Highland Ability Battery.
- The Ball Foundation produces the Ball Aptitude Battery.
- Aptitude Inventory Measurement Service produces the AIMS Aptitude Battery.

Attitude and Interest: Concept and Measurement

The concept of *attitude* occupies a very favoured position in social psychology. Psychologists as well informed as G. Allport (1) and G. Murphy (9) consider it the central concept in the field; various textbooks have indicated its usefulness in the advance of the science; and the literature revolving around "attitudes" has grown in the past 20 years to voluminous proportions. Yet the concept, despite its key position, is marked by considerable confusion.

Diversity of Definitions

Examination of the various definitions and discussions of attitude offered by social psychologists, for example, reveals that there is an amazing diversity of conceptions of what the term denotes. The range of these views can be illustrated by noting the following dissimilar definitions of attitude:

A person's attitude is "the relatively stable overt behaviour which affects his status" (3).

When a certain type of experience is constantly repeated a change of set is brought about which affects many central neurons and tends to spread over other parts of the central nervous system. These changes in the general set of the central nervous system temper the process of reception; they lead to the formation of certain general modes of receiving and integrating stimuli. In terms of the subjective life these general sets are called attitudes (15).

Attitudes in the narrow and more specific sense are essentially motor sets of the organism toward some specific or general stimulus. They rest upon innate stimulus-response patterns as these have become modified, elaborated, and integrated through learning in the social world.... Attitudes do not exist without reference to value meanings. And meanings are related to situations of all sorts around which we have constructed our habits and built up a series of images (16).

An attitude is "a process of individual consciousness which determines real or possible activity of the individual in the social world" (13).

The first definition refers to a particular kind of overt behaviour. The (330) second points to a kind of neurological action. The third includes both neurological action and action that involves meaning, imagery, and value. The fourth definition points to any process of individual consciousness. These four views of attitude suggest the extent to which conceptions of the attitude differ. The published writings of psychologists show no general agreement upon what the term attitude denotes.

Divergent Theoretical Functions of the Concept

While it is a perfectly legitimate scientific procedure to define terms in any, manner one wishes, the fact that a single psychological concept should be conceived in such dissimilar ways by social psychologists indicates the state of confusion in the use of the term. How is it that a single "concept" has so many different meanings?

Probably the answer lies in the different roles which the concept plays within the different psychological schemes of various psychological theorists. The concept has been gradually taken over by divergent approaches within the field. Despite the clashing methodological implications resident in some of these approaches, various social psychologists have been able to use the term because they have assigned to it quite different roles.

To illustrate what is meant by this contention, one can point to the different fashions in which the concept has been utilized by such writers as Thomas (13), Park (10), Dewey (6), and Bain (3). Thomas' concept of attitude afforded him the subjective factor with which—together with the objective factor (value)—he sought to account for human social behaviour. Thomas was looking for causal explanation and believed it could not' be found without taking into account both objective and subjective factors. The "attitude" supplied the necessary subjective tool which enabled him to seek laws of social behaviour. On the other hand Park used the attitude for a different purpose. He sought the ultimate social forces within each individual which would account for all human behaviour. He employed attitudes as these ultimate units of analysis. In contrast, Dewey built his social psychological scheme for the analysis of human behaviour upon three analytic tools: impulse, attitude, and thought. Attitude organizes impulse in this scheme, and must be taken into account in order to understand human behaviour; one must realize the importance of the reaction of attitude to impulse and thought. Bain's use of the attitude differs strikingly from each of the above. He wrote as a strict behaviourist, holding that subjective states are illusions and that their use in analysis of behaviour is harmful to the advance of social science. Hence Bain employed the attitude to refer (331) to a particular kind of overt behaviour, for it is overt behaviour which is the only legitimate phenomenon for research study.

Each of these four theorists makes his concept of attitude perform some special function within his particular psychological scheme. These functions assigned the concept are not identical, and this taken in wider application is the probable explanation for the exceedingly dissimilar conceptions of the attitude held by various social psychologists. Any one term used to cover such different phenomena could hardly refer to the same or even similar referents. Because the psychological schemes employed by various theorists arc so diverse, and because the word "attitude" is used to refer to some structure in each of these schemes, it is unlikely that there could be general agreement on the meaning of the concept.

Empirically Ungrounded Character of Attitude Theory

If this is so it suggests that definitions of the attitude are not generally grounded upon nor derived from empirical research. It seems unlikely that the concept (or concepts) arose during and as a direct result of the solving of empirical problems. That attitude theory is indeed largely ungrounded can be established by pointing to: (a) the paucity of verified knowledge about the nature of attitudes, and (b) the inclusion in many definitions of the attitude of conceptions which are unfounded or unverified.

Examination of the literature of attitude research indicates that although there is a very sizeable amount of research which turns about the concept, there is very little research which has been concerned with the study of the attitude as such.

Study of attitudes as attitudes, i.e., the "nature" of attitudes-would be expected to yield knowledge concerning such problems as: how attitudes are formed, how they are changed, how they disappear, how they are related to personal organization, and how they influence behaviour subsequent to their formation.

One would expect to find the cumulative results of research concerning such problems summarized in the textbooks and theoretical literature. Such summaries, however, are almost totally lacking. What little there is likely to take the form of statements sometimes platitudinous, sometimes of doubtful validity, and practically never based upon any rigorous empirical research. (332) The emission of research conclusions from textbooks and theoretical literature reflects the marked neglect by research of the important problem of the nature of attitudes. In the literature of research there are very few reports devoted to the study of attitudes as attitudes. Students of research do not seem to be directly concerned with the problem. As a result of this neglect, social psychological research seems to have very little to report with regard to the nature of attitudes.

This paucity of verified knowledge points to the generally unfounded or unverified character of contemporary attitude theory. In view of the fact that verified knowledge is so meager, it is unlikely that the various definitions of attitude offered in the literature can be composed of more than unfounded or unverified hypotheses.

It is possible to point, in fact, to several conceptions or views implied in definitions of attitude, which are unfounded or unverified. For example, a number of social psychologists view attitudes as having always a rather fixed and settled character. They ignore so completely the possibility of rapid change of attitudes that stability is made to appear an essential feature of all attitudes (5, 8, 12, 14).

Another questionable conception of the attitude is that which views the attitude as a psychological element; that is, as a basic unit for use in scientific causal analysis. There are some psychologists who think of the attitude as an element which can be employed in causal analysis in much the same fashion as chemical and physical elements are used in unraveling chemical and physical causations (2, 10, 13, 11). In the scheme of causal analysis which employs the notion of "clement," one seeks to explain the occurrence of an event by describing the "interaction" of elements. The method consists essentially in analyzing the event which sets the problem into constituent elements, and then explaining this event by describing the relationships which hold between the elements. This conception when carried over to the attitude is not based upon actual fact: nowhere in the literature has the author found an instance of the attitude used as a genuine psychological element in unraveling causation. Attitudes, it is true, are used to "explain" behaviour in the same sense that common sense explains behaviour-"His attitude of curiosity prompted him to go to the window"-but this is not genuine causal explanation as the older sciences know it. And since the concept is not today used as a psychological element, the view that conceives of the attitude as an element is based upon an erroneous conception of the attitude's function in actual research.

A third questionable conception implied in many definitions of the attitude (333) is that which think of the attitude as a specific psychological concept, different from and exclusive of other established psychological concepts. Various psychologists have distinguished, for example, between "attitude" and concepts such a "interest," "wish," "belief," "desire," "impulse" (1, 6. 4, 7). By distinguishing the attitude from other psychological categories various students have indicated that attitudes-are not to be identified or confused with wishes, impulses, opinions, and the like. Actually this differentiation of the attitudes front other concepts is unwarranted. An examination of the actual concrete use of the term by local psychologists-theorists and research students alike-shows very clearly that attitudes are not distinct and apart from wishes, desires, beliefs; rather sonic attitudes can be pointed to as wishes, some as impulses, sonic as opinions, some as beliefs. In fact the number of kinds of psychological terms under which different attitudes can he classified is very great: tile limit depends apparently upon the limits of one's psychological vocabulary-impulse, plan, demand, desire, decision, belief, faith, preference, wish, urge, tendency, longing, hunger, general perspective, philosophy of life, outlook, and so on. Consequently the attempt to set up the attitude as a concept independent of such concepts as the above does not seem justifiable.

The fact that these three views briefly discussed above are questionable indicates the non-empirical character of definitions in which these views are incorporated. Since these unverified views arc shared by various social psychologists, they constitute further evidence that many definitions of the attitude are not empirically grounded.

Divorce of Attitude Research from Attitude Theory

This in turn suggests that research employing the concept is not effectively guided by attitude theory. That there exists this relative divorce of research and theory can be demonstrated.

In the first place students rarely state in their research reports any definition of attitude which guided their investigations. This omission suggests strongly that this research, although employing the concept of attitude, is not linked with attitude theory. It is probable that if definitions formulated by psychological theorists served to guide research then investigators would riot take the concept for granted, so to speak, in their researches.

Moreover, examination of these research reports yields no evidence that special formulations of the attitude usually guide research.

The validity of this assertion can be made more convincing than its bare assertion by noting the different manner with which theorists and research (334) students treat attitudinal causation. Practically every psychologist who has defined the attitude has conceived of the attitude as entering into the causation of behaviour. Attitudes are thought to lie behind and "precipitate," "determine," "condition," or "cause" overt behaviour. Since attitudes are so generally conceived to enter into the causation of behaviour one would expect to find this conception guiding research. Use of the attitude to unravel the causation of behaviour should be frequent in empirical inquiries.

That research students use the notion of attitude to explain behaviour is apparent even in a casual survey. However this research use of attitudes to account for causation is a common sense rather than a technical procedure. It bears no closer relation to scientific causation than does common sense "explaining" in general. Common sense explanation is a device for setting behaviour into an understandable context; for finding "reasons" which account plausibly for the act; for predicting behaviour by means of judging how a person feels about certain objects. Common sense explanation is not genuine causal explanation. There is no effort to formulate a closed system of forces in such *a way* that reciprocal influences resulting in an effect can be accurately determined and rigorously checked.

The fact that psychological research does not use attitudes to explain behaviour in a genuine causative fashion is additional indication of the divorce of research from attitude theory. Practically every theoretical formulation of the concept states that the attitude enters into the causation of human acts. Yet research derives so little guidance from these theoretical formulations that it does not—or cannot—use the concept to genuinely explain human acts.

Identity of Technical Concept with Common Sense Notion

If research employing the concept of attitude is not intimately linked with attitude theory, the question arises: what then is the character of the concept which *is* being used by research students? An answer is that the research concept of attitude is not a technical psychological concept but a common sense concept. Students are employing the same concept of attitude that is in everyday lay use. This identity of research and lay concepts can be demonstrated by noting that students in reporting research invariably use the *word* attitude in a fashion identical with the common ordinary use of the word. Examples taken at random from research literature differ in no way from examples chosen at random from lay sources. Indeed, in view of the divorce of (335) attitude theory from research and the meagerness of verified knowledge about attitudes, it seems very unlikely that research students could be employing anything other than a common sense concept.

Usefulness of Concept

The fact that psychologists are using a lap concept in their research poses the problem of "usefulness." Is it possible that the research use of a concept as imprecise and naive as this commonsense notion of "attitude" must necessarily he can eventuate in valuable results? Are psychologists correct in believing that the attitude is exceedingly useful?

We have noted that psychologists are not concerned generally with studying the referent of "attitude" as such. Rather, psychologists use attitudes as instruments for studying something else in which they are interested. They use attitudes as tools for studying various areas of social life—such as the organization of groups, relations between groups, organization of personalities, and relations between persons. In the study of these areas of social life, the concept of attitude is used as a device for gaining an understanding of the specific subject tinder investigation. By looking for and observing attitudes, or by correlating attitudes with some category, the investigator is enabled to lean something about the organization of the group or persons being studied and the, relations between it' and other groups (or persons). It is almost certainly because the concept is such a convenient device for the study of diverse areas of social life that the attitude is held by psychologists to be such a useful tool for research.

The convenient and useful character of the attitude can be accounted for also upon somewhat different grounds.

In the first place the concept is used in an over-all fashion to refer to a great number of diverse "inner" psychological activities: wishing, desiring, wanting, believing, demanding, being interested in, deciding, realizing, and so forth. These psychological activities go on in many of the areas of human behaviour which interest psychologists. Consequently this sprawling concept of attitude serves to focus inquiry upon various forms of "inner" psychological behaviour without the necessity of psychologists having to make clear what particular kind of psychological activity they are dealing with at any specific time.

The word "attitude" is, in fact, so convenient that it can be used usually without designating what kind of activity it refers to other than the presumed one of "having an attitude." (336) In the second place the term "attitude" provides students with a convenient labelling device whereby they can depict or describe psychological activities in very short hand fashion. Such phrases as: a clinging attitude; a vindictive and almost cruel attitude; a very sentimental and affectionate attitude-these point very concisely to relationships between a person and an object. Similarly attitudes can also be used as labels in conjunction with extended adjective and descriptive phrases to demarcate rather subtlety one or more psychological activity.

Finally psychologists with very different backgrounds and schemes of interpretation can use the notion of attitude because attitudes cannot be seen, because attitudes are internal and have to be interpreted from external acts and gestures. Thus an observer interested in class structure may interpret various acts as being expressive of attitudes like class-conscious attitudes or attitudes typical of some given social class. An observer of human behaviour who is interested in personal relations is likely to detect attitudes more like: an attitude of uncritical adulation, or, a very sentimental and affectionate attitude. Similarly attitudes expressed by acts can be interpreted (and libelled) psychiatrical or psychoanalytically or anthropologically.

These are ways in which overt acts can be interpreted and the "underlying" attitude inferred. It is no Wonder then that psychologists, though adhering to different' (and often conflicted) schemes of interpreting behaviour, can use the notion of attitude and find it a useful instrument in inquiry.

A Suggested Method for Refining Tile Research Concept

In the light of the role which the concept of attitude plays in research its convenient and useful character can scarcely be denied. It is important to remember, however, that while this concept serves as a convenient tool it is nevertheless a common sense concept.

It follows that students engaged in research involving the concept arc using an extremely crude instrument. Common sense concepts are notoriously vague, unrefined, and imprecise. However valuable they may be for lay purposes they are not formulated neatly enough for scientific use. Scientific inquiry demands concepts whose referents can be clearly denoted and isolated.

The use of the common sense concept of attitude by psychologists is probably equivalent to chemists using the common sense (17th century) concept of "burning" to study chemical behaviour, or physicists using such crude notions as "speed" to study physical behaviour. (337) It would seems clear that as long as social psychologists rely upon a concept which is no more definitive, refined, and sophisticated than that same concept as it is used by laymen, then research involving the concept is going to be handicapped.

The question arises: if research is handicapped because of the employment of a crude concept, and yet one does not wish to discard that concept because it performs a seemingly worthwhile function, how can it be rendered more precise and scientifically usable? The crudity *of* the attitude and its usefulness together make evident the need for critical revision of the concept.

One path by which this objective might be attained is suggested by the identity of the common sense usage and the research usage of the word "attitude." One might study the usage of the word in common ordinary discourse to see if it is possible to isolate the referent (or referents, perhaps) to which this usage points. By careful examination, analysis, and comparison of uses, it might lie possible to discover some solid "core" (or cores) which is pointed to etch time the word is used.

If one could discover an identical referent pointed to by each use of the word, lie would be on the road to making the concept more precise, definite, tangible, sophisticated, and consequently more scientifically usable. Moreover, one could expect as a result of this effort to discover additional leads toward the further refining of this referent.

This kind of referent analysis could go hand in hand with intimate study of concrete human behaviour. Such study would be expected to yield clues relevant to the study of attitudes qua attitudes. Hypotheses could then be raised about the nature of the attitude which in turn could be checked empirically by careful study of human behaviour.

An example of Ions-such interaction between empirical data; nut attitude analysis might be carried on is suggested by such a notion as: attitudes which arc linked intimately with the personality organization are much more resistant to change than are those attitudes which see more peripheral to the personality organization. There might be two "types" of attitudes and attitude change. Concrete empirical study might verify or invalidate this statement about attitudes; the notion of attitude might tints lie refined, and he brought to bear again upon further empirical study of attitudes.

In this way uric might expect to attitude, eventually, some knowledge about the phenomena pointed to by the term "attitude" and thereby trace the relations between attitude and other psychological phenomena. One might (338) hope also to get the working relation between theory and research that does not exist today.

Integrated Personality

Well integrated personality is the sum total of harmonious expression of:

1. Physical self
2. Energy self
3. Intellectual self
4. Mental self
5. Blissful self.

Physical self relates to our senses. Proper nourishment and growth of physical faculties is essential by way of balanced diet, recreation, music, care and concern from near & dear ones. Mind & body are related. A simple pat on the back for any achievement in life goes a long way to build up confidence. However discretion and discrimination are the key words in this regard, otherwise, there will be chances that senses would create havoc by way of infatuation and attachment to the sense objects.

Energy self is subtler than the first. It relates to metabolism and gross manifestation of energy (PRANA) e.g breathing. The control of prana is achieved by control of anger, anxiety, and restlessness.

Intellectual self concern with discriminative power and knowledge, what we call *Buddhi*. In addition to sincere and formal studies reading of books like biographies of noble person.

Mental self is related to stress and psychology. Here selflessness, control, concentration, and calmness play an essential role.

Anandamaya Kosh or **Blissful self** is the function of state of being. It calls for remaining calm and unaffected nay to remain happy, free from worldly affair, in calamities and disasters, in suffering or loss, in failure and success.

To attain these five fold method, we follow:

1. Self effort
2. Self control
3. Self reliance
4. Self sacrifice
5. Self knowledge

Swami Vivekananda says that IP is but the aggregate of our tendencies, the sum total of the bent of mind. We are what our thoughts made us. Thoughts travel far & fast. So take care of thoughts. If good impression prevails, the IP becomes good. An integrated person develops upward. We are influenced by:

Influence of Parents: The personality begins to get formed in prenatal stage. Parents knowingly or unknowingly mould the personality of the child by their thoughts and actions. When the child is little big, he watches and imitates his parents. Mother influences in moulding the character of a child. Saints are generally born of men and women of great character. For building IP earlier, it is better we catch our children early.

Influence of teacher: Teachers influence in moulding the IP of children. If parents and teachers are confirmed noble character, their wards will mostly be of same character. That is why, education in olden days was in the hand of ideal man and sages.

Influence of environment: Besides parents and teachers, there is a powerful influence of social environment. This can be creatively handled for building character only through homes. Ethical conducts have to be cultivated from childhood which takes care of the human personality and its fulfilment. Success lies in the development of will power, character, concentration, detachment, righteousness, ethics and attainment of spiritual illumination.

Unit-IX

Mental Health and Hygiene

Concept of Mental Health and Hygiene

Mental Health

Mental health is a term used to describe either a level of cognitive or emotional well-being or an absence of a mental disorder. From perspectives of the discipline of positive psychology or holism mental health may include an individual's ability to enjoy life and procure a balance between life activities and efforts to achieve psychological resilience.

The World Health Organization defines mental health as ""a state of well-being in which the individual realizes his or her own abilities, can cope with the normal stresses of life, can work productively and fruitfully, and is able to make a contribution to his or her community." It was previously stated that there was no one "official" definition of mental health. Cultural differences, subjective assessments, and competing professional theories all affect how "mental health" is defined.

History

In the mid-19th century, William Sweetzer was the first to clearly define the term "mental hygiene", which can be seen as the precurser to contemporary approaches to work on promoting positive mental health. Isaac Ray, one of thirteen founders of the American Psychiatric Association, further defined mental hygiene as an art to preserve the mind against incidents and influences which would inhibit or destroy its energy, quality or development.

At the beginning of the 20th century, Clifford Beers founded the National Committee for Mental Hygiene and opened the first outpatient mental health clinic in the United States.

Perspectives

Mental Wellbeing

Mental health can be seen as a continuum, where an individual's mental health may have many different possible values. Mental wellness is generally viewed as a positive attribute, such that a person can reach enhanced levels of mental health, even if they do not have any diagnosable mental health condition. This definition of mental health highlights emotional well-being, the capacity to live a full and creative life, and the flexibility to deal with life's inevitable challenges. Many therapeutic systems and self-help books offer methods and philosophies espousing strategies and techniques vaunted as effective for further improving the mental wellness of otherwise healthy people. Positive psychology is increasingly prominent in mental health. A holistic model of mental health generally includes concepts based upon anthropological, educational, psychological, religious and sociological perspectives, as well as theoretical perspectives from personality, social, clinical, health and developmental psychology. An example of a wellness model includes one developed by Myers, Sweeny and Witmer. It includes five life tasks — essence or spirituality, work and leisure, friendship, love and self-direction—and twelve sub tasks—sense of worth, sense of control, realistic beliefs, emotional awareness and coping, problem solving and creativity, sense of humour, nutrition, exercise, self care, stress management, gender identity, and cultural identity—are identified as characteristics of healthy functioning and a major component of wellness. The components provide a means of responding to the circumstances of life in a manner that promotes healthy functioning. Most of the US Population is not educated on Mental Health.

Lack of a Mental Disorder

Mental health can also be defined as an absence of a major mental health condition (for example, one of the diagnoses in the Diagnostic and Statistical Manual, IV) though recent evidence stemming from positive psychology suggests mental health is more than the mere absence of a mental disorder or illness. Therefore the impact of social, cultural, physical and education can all affect someone's mental health.

Cultural and Religious Considerations

Mental health can be socially constructed and socially defined; that is, different professions, communities, societies and cultures have very different ways of conceptualizing its nature and causes, determining what is mentally healthy, and deciding what interventions are appropriate. Thus, different professionals will have different cultural and religious backgrounds and experiences, which may impact the methodology applied during treatment.

Many mental health professionals are beginning to, or already understand, the importance of competency in religious diversity and spirituality. The American Psychological Association explicitly states that religion must be respected. Education in spiritual and religious matters is also required by the American Psychiatric Association.

Mental Hygiene

The science of maintaining mental health and preventing the development of psychosis, neurosis, or other mental disorders. Since the founding of the United Nations the concepts of mental health and hygiene have achieved international acceptance. As defined in the 1946 constitution of the World Health Organization, "health is a state of complete physical, mental, and social well-being, and not merely the absence of disease or infirmity." The term mental health represents a variety of human aspirations: rehabilitation of the mentally disturbed, prevention of mental disorder, reduction of tension in a stressful world, and attainment of a state of well-being in which the individual functions at a level consistent with his or her mental potential. As noted by the World Federation for Mental Health, the concept of optimum mental health refers not to an absolute or ideal state but to the best possible state insofar as circumstances are alterable. Mental health is regarded as a condition of the individual, relative to the capacities and social-environmental context of that person. Mental hygiene includes all measures taken to promote and to preserve mental health. Community mental health refers to the extent to which the organization and functioning of the community determines, or is conducive to, the mental health of its members.

Throughout the ages the mentally disturbed have been viewed with a mixture of fear and revulsion. Their fate generally has been one of rejection, neglect, and ill treatment. Though in ancient medical writings there are references to mental disturbance that display views very similar to modern humane attitudes, interspersed in the same literature are instances of socially sanctioned cruelty based upon the belief that mental disorders have supernatural origins such as demonic possession.

Even reformers sometimes used harsh methods of treatment; for example, the 18th-century American physician Benjamin Rush endorsed the practice of restraining mental patients with his notorious "tranquilising chair."

Concept of Mental Health

The concept of mental health, given its polysemic nature and its imprecise borders, benefits from a historical perspective to be better understood. What today is broadly understood by "mental health" can have its origins tracked back to developments in public health, in clinical psychiatry and in other branches of knowledge.

Although references to mental health as a state can be found in the English language well before the 20th century, technical references to mental health as a field or discipline are not found before 1946. During that year, the International Health Conference, held in New York, decided to establish the World Health Organization (WHO) and a Mental Health Association was founded in London. Before that date, found are references to the corresponding concept of "mental hygiene", which first appeared in the English literature in 1843, in a book entitled Mental hygiene or an examination of the intellect and passions designed to illustrate their influence on health and duration of life 1. Moreover, in 1849, "healthy mental and physical development of the citizen" had already been included as the first objective of public health in a draft law submitted to the Berlin Society of Physicians and Surgeons 2.

In 1948, the WHO was created and in the same year the first International Congress on Mental Health took place in London. At the second session of the WHO's Expert Committee on Mental Health (September 11-16, 1950), "mental health" and "mental hygiene" were defined as follows 3: "Mental hygiene refers to all the activities and techniques which encourage and maintain mental health.

Mental health is a condition, subject to fluctuations due to biological and social factors, which enables the individual to achieve a satisfactory synthesis of his own potentially conflicting, instinctive drives; to form and maintain harmonious relations with others; and to participate in constructive changes in his social and physical environment."

However, a clear and widely accepted definition of mental health as a discipline was (and is) still missing. Significantly, the Dorland's Medical Dictionary does not carry an entry on mental health, whereas the Campbell's Dictionary of Psychiatry gives it two meanings: first, as a synonym of mental hygiene and second, as a state of psychological wellbeing. The Oxford English Dictionary defines mental hygiene as a set of measures to preserve mental health, and later refers to mental health as a state. These lexicographic concepts nonetheless, more and more mental health is employed in the sense of a discipline (e.g., sections/divisions in health ministries or secretaries, or departments in universities), with an almost perfect replacement of mental hygiene.

In addition, given this polysemic nature of mental health, its delimitation in relation to psychiatry (understood as the medical specialty concerned with the study, prevention, diagnosis and treatment of mental disorders or diseases) is not always clear. There is a more or less widespread effort to set mental health at least aside from psychiatry and at most as an overarching concept with encompasses psychiatry.

The Origins of Mental Health

The Mental Hygiene Movement

The origin of the mental hygiene movement can be attributed to the work of Clifford Beers in the USA. In 1908 he published A mind that found itself 4, a book based on his personal experience of admissions to three mental hospitals. The book had a great repercussion and in the same year a Mental Hygiene Society was established in Connecticut. The term "mental hygiene" had been suggested to Beers by Adolf Meyer 5 and enjoyed a quick popularity thanks to the creation in 1909 of the National Commission of Mental Hygiene. From 1919 onwards, the internationalization of activities of this Commission led to the establishment of some national associations concerned with mental hygiene: in France 6 and South Africa 7 in 1920, in Italy 8 and Hungary 9 in 1924. From these national associations the International Committee on Mental Hygiene was created and later superseded by the World Federation of Mental Health.

The mental hygiene movement, in its origins and reflecting Beers' experience in mental hospitals, was primarily and basically concerned with the improvement of the care of people with mental disorders. In Beers' own words: "When the National Committee was organized, in 1909, its chief concern was to humanize the care of the insane: to eradicate the abuses, brutalities and neglect from which the mentally sick have traditionally suffered."

It was at a later stage that the Committee enlarged its program to include the "milder forms of mental disability" and a greater concern with preventive work. The rationale behind this shift was the belief that "mental disorders frequently have their beginnings in childhood and youth and that preventive measures are most effective in early life", and that environmental conditions and modes of living produce mental ill health.

By 1937, the US National Committee for Mental Hygiene stated that it sought to achieve its purposes by: a) promoting early diagnosis and treatment; b) developing adequate hospitalization; c) stimulating research; d) securing public understanding and support of psychiatric and mental hygiene activities; e) instructing individuals and groups in the personal application of mental hygiene principles; and f) cooperating with governmental and private agencies whose work touches at any point the field of mental hygiene.

Thus, the mental hygiene movement had initially a para-psychiatric nature, directing its efforts towards the improvement of psychiatric care. The inclusion of preventive activities among its interests did not distinguish it from psychiatry: the movement aimed at maximizing what was accepted and proposed by the most advanced psychiatrists of the epoch in the USA, most of whom followed a psychoanalytical orientation.

According to the group which launched it, the mental hygiene movement "visualized, not a single patient, but a whole community; and it considered each member of that community as an individual whose mental and emotional status was determined by definite causative factors and whose compelling need was for prevention rather than cure. The Mental Hygiene Movement, then, bears the same relation to psychiatry that the public-health movement, of which it forms a part, bears to medicine in general. It is an organized community response to a recognized community need." 4. On the other hand, it was also stated that: "At the present time both psychiatrists and mental hygienists are more than ever conscious that their objectives are in fact identical and that each group needs the other for the fulfilment of their common task." 4.

The World Health Organization

From its very beginning, the WHO has always had an administrative section specially dedicated to mental health, as an answer to requests from its Member States. The first Report of the WHO's Director General 10, in its English version, refers to an administrative section called "Mental Health". However, the French version of the same report calls it "Hygiene Mentale". Well until the 1960s we find hygiene as the French translation of health in some WHO publications and in some instances we find also mental hygiene used interchangeably with mental health in the English version of some documents. In the preamble to the WHO Constitutions, it was stated that "health is a state of complete physical, mental and social wellbeing and not merely the absence of disease or infirmity" 14, a now widely quoted definition. This definition is clearly a holistic one, intended to overcome the old dichotomies of body vs. mind and physical vs. psychic. It is also a pragmatic one, insofar as it incorporates into medicine a social dimension, gradually developed in Europe during the 19th century.

It should be noted that mental, in WHO's definition of health (as well as physical and social) refers to dimensions of a state and not to a specific domain or discipline. Therefore, according to this concept, it is incongruous to refer to physical health, mental health or social health. Should one wish to specify a particular dimension, the most appropriate noun to designate it should be wellbeing and not health (e.g., mental wellbeing or social wellbeing). This negligent use of the word health seems to have been also in operation when mental hygiene (a social movement, or a domain of activity) was replaced by mental health (originally intended to designate a state and later transformed in a particular domain or field of activity).

The International Congress of Mental Health

The First International Congress of Mental Health was organized in London by the British National Association for Mental Hygiene from 16 to 21 August, 1948. Starting as an International Conference on Mental Hygiene, it ended with a series of recommendations on mental health. Throughout the proceedings of the conference, hygiene and health, qualifying mental, are used interchangeably, sometimes in the same paragraph, without any clear conceptual distinction. However, in the 17 pages of the recommendations of the conference, hygiene is very sparingly used. At the end of the congress, the International Committee on Mental Hygiene was superseded by the World Federation for Mental Health.

In addition to the wording employed in the proceedings of that congress, gradually replacing hygiene by health, some of its recommendations were also influential at other levels. An example is recommendation 6 to the WHO that "as soon as practicable, an advisory expert committee be established, composed of professional personnel in the field of mental health and human relations".

The conference had been convened under the theme "Mental Health and World Citizenship". From a conceptual point of view, nevertheless, and perhaps reflecting an immediately post-war situation, discussions over world citizenship prevailed over those on mental health. Only one concept of mental health was put forward, by J.C. Flugel, Chairman of the Conference's Programme Committee: "Mental health is regarded as a condition which permits the optimal development, physical, intellectual and emotional, of the individual, so far as this is compatible with that of other individuals." 15. Echoing concerns about the absence, or rather limited number of, participants from places such as Far East, South America and the Soviet Union, the hope was expressed that "mental health as understood in Western countries [is not] necessarily at variance with the sense in which it is understood in other countries" 15.

In a more detailed way, some delegates elaborated on what was summarized as the "four levels of mental health work: custodial, therapeutic, preventive and positive" 15. It is not difficult to see a considerable overlapping between this proposal and the one already implemented by the mental hygiene movement.

At the closing session, O.L. Forel, Lecturer in Psychiatry at the University of Geneva, answering to criticisms that mental hygiene, as understood in that conference, went beyond the medical and scientific framework, made a clearly political (in Plato's sense) statement by saying that: "I dare hope to be your interpreter in expressing our pride that so many scientists came here not at all to develop their respective sciences, but to have them at men's service" 15.

Reading through the proceedings of this congress gives one a feeling of the tensions between a pragmatic approach, developed by the mental hygiene movement (basically defended by delegates from the USA), and a more politically-oriented approach, proposed by other participants, perhaps translating the experiences of some delegates from European countries, which had severely suffered from the war. In the end this latter approach prevailed, with the transformation of the mental hygiene movement into the mental health movement. Perhaps as a reflection of this basically political movement, in 1949 the National Institute of Mental Health started its activities in the USA.

Recent Developments

After half a century of the mental health, and almost a century of the mental hygiene movements, some developments can be perceived. On a more general level, the WHO's very concept of health has been recently questioned; formulated half a century ago, it is no longer felt by some as much appropriate to the current situation 16,17.

On the whole, mental health continues to be used both to designate a state, a dimension of health – an essential element in the definition of health – and to refer to the movement derived from the mental hygiene movement, corresponding to the application of psychiatry to groups, communities and societies, rather than on an individual basis, as is the case with clinical psychiatry. However, mental health is, quite unfortunately, still viewed by many as a discipline, either as a synonym of psychiatry, or as one of its complementary fields.

A recent trend has been the addition of the qualifier public to either mental health or to psychiatry, as it can be seen in a WHO document entitled Public mental health 18, or in a journal named Psiquiatria Publica, published in Spain since 1989. This is very much in line with the concept of mental health as a movement rather than a discipline.

In 2001, the WHO dedicated its annual report (The World Health Report-Mental health: new knowledge, new hope) to mental health 19. In that same year, the theme of the World Health Day was Stop Exclusion – Dare to Care, a quite clear political statement, that I am sure would have immensely pleased Clifford Beers.

In the message from the WHO Director-General that opens that report, Gro H. Brundtland summarizes the three main knowledge areas covered by the document: a) effectiveness of prevention and treatment, b) service planning and provision, and c) policies to break down stigma and discrimination and adequate funds for prevention and treatment. If one allows for the semantic variations between the beginnings of the 20th and the 21st centuries, the same concerns of the origins of the mental hygiene movement, discussed earlier on, can be found in the mental health content of the World Health Report. Perhaps the biggest difference between these two political platforms is the emphasis on the improvement of hospital care in the former (the only form of treatment available by then), and the contemporary emphasis on distancing mental health from psychiatric hospitals and placing it in the community.

However, one must admit that, unfortunately, what was high in Beers' agenda in 1909, namely, an improvement in the standards of mental health care and an eradication of the abuses to which people with mental disorders are usually subject, is still a major concern of the most progressive and advanced agenda of people interested in the promotion of mental health around the world.

Onflict and Frustration

Some scientific studies clearly indicated that the feelings of continual conflict and frustration will have a negative effect upon our well-being. The chronic inability to be successful, meet one's goals, or even know one's goals is weakened. Unhappiness, frustration and unresolved needs and desires cause great emotional unhappiness.

The conflict and frustration may be on a conscious level or subconscious level. There may often be conflict in our emotions and attitudes between the conscious and the subconscious mind. For example, an individual may appear to be calm and happy, yet underneath that mask of calmness could be repressed anger and hurt that is hidden. A shy person may actually be full of rage.

The individual tries to maintain his or her life in a way that keeps the mask of the calm person or shy person in place. When there is conflict, and the person cannot predict and be secure in his or her world, then there may be fear and pain for the individual. He or she may not be able to cope. When there is too much conflict between the conscious and subconscious mind, disease may occur, and other emotional problems may appear. Therefore, always be calm and collective in most problems of life and try to face them head on with full determination.

Frustration

We strive to gratify our wants and desires, our goals, aims, and ambitions. Introspection and self-knowledge make this much self-evident; experience with others confirms the generalization.

Moreover, we are often unable to satisfy our desires or accomplish our goals. Sometimes our ambitions exceed our abilities, or we misperceive the possibilities. But sometimes we are blocked by an external barrier that precludes gratification. This may be a traffic jam preventing us from reaching an appointment, a college rule prohibiting us from taking a particular course, an amorous neighbourhood tom cat interrupting our sleep, or our race restricting professional advancement. Whatever the barrier, we are frustrated. All of us are so frustrated from time to time.

In addition, we all have experienced irritation and anger at some frustrations. A long line preventing us from seeing an eagerly awaited movie, a crush of shoppers hindering the purchase of some simple necessities, a slow driver obstructing a narrow road, probably have aroused in all of us that familiar flush of annoyance, even anger. That frustration of our desires and goals occasionally leads to anger is a commonplace. It is subjectively unquestionable—a fact of our existence.

Of course, not all frustrations lead to anger. Indeed, it is more common to accept frustration—the blockage of our wants or goals—as feedback suggesting that we adjust or alter our aims. We do this automatically, hour by hour, day by day. Frustration signals the error in the trial-and-error process by which we dialectically adjust our perspectives to external powers and potentialities. To live, to assert oneself, is to be hindered, to face difficulties, to be *opposed*. My desire to write this section uninterruptedly is hindered by construction noise in the background; my desire for physical comfort is defeated by the summer heat; my search for the right words to express my "understanding" is blocked by the barrier between structured language and unstructured "insight" and feelings.

Moreover, when I let my consciousness stroll through the nested levels of my existence, I am also aware of a multitude of frustrations that reach consciousness like a flock of pheasants startled out of tall grass. Frustrations associated with family, research, teaching, politics, and the growing structure of coercive rules and laws. As I write, my life is within a matrix of such frustrations, high and low, large and small, significant and trivial.

Yet at the moment I am content, relatively happy, and feel no irritation, no anger.

Besides our desires and goals, our frustrations and anger, there are two other commonplace facts of life. We sometimes desire or aim to injure or hurt others, and behave in such a manner, sometimes because of our frustrations. Again, in our subjective world, these two facts are incontestable. Our awareness of them enables us to better perceive others to adjust our interests and interactions, and to develop predictive expectations. We can then understand why on a hot day in slow city traffic, one motorist will attack another for blocking his path, why a parent whose losing bridge game is interrupted for the fifth time by a child will vigorously spank him, and why a mistress cast off by her lover will send poison pen letters to his wife.

In the late 1930s, the commonplace enabling us to understand such behaviour in certain contexts was erected into an invariant law of nature by a group of Yale psychologists (Dollard et al., 1939). First, they equated aggression with the desire to hurt or injure others. This effectively confused the various forms of aggression with one overt manifestation and confounded the bases of aiming to harm another, which may be instrumental (as in spanking a child), defensive (as in kicking an attacker), or hostile (as in spreading malicious gossip). Were one to equate love with kissing, the conceptual, cognitive confusion would be no less.

Second, frustration was defined as interference with a goal *response,* thus keying frustration to an objective barrier or difficulty, and to manifest behaviour. Interference was felt to be through punishment or goal inaccessibility, further confusing frustration as blockage with frustration as deprivation.

Conflict Helix

The relationship of relative deprivation-turned-injustice vector to the process of conflict is easily clarified. Injustice vectors—the moral sense of deprivation relative to others—are part of the conflict situation. These are vectors of interest, the opposition of which creates the conflict situation. Here, awareness (or perception) and the situation give context and meaning to the opposing interests; expectations of Behavioural outcomes interrelate the injustice vector and its drive to action with the capability of the other and our expectation of his behaviour. In other words, the situation of conflict involves our interests and their justness; our perception of others and our sense of injustice by comparison; and our beliefs about the capabil'ties of others and the outcomes of our actions. Within the framework of the helix, the conflict situation comprises the variables important to transforming the potential for collective violence into the potential for class violence and, finally, into manifest violence. At the collective level, the injustice vector fundamentally defines the class consciousness necessary to the class struggle within all organizations, including the state.

The initiation phase of manifest conflict involves a trigger provoking the will to action, and the occurrence of such a mechanism depends on the balance of powers an individual perceives between himself and others. Consequently a sense of injustice is no guarantee of action. This is also true of Gurr's model, in which the transformation of potential to manifestation depends on a balance of powers.

But deprivation theory does not explain what happens after the manifest conflict or violence ensues, while the conflict helix is in mid-ascent. Out of manifest conflict a balance is formed among the diverse interests held by people on the basis of their capability and wills. There ensues adjustment among the diverse vectors of injustice, an adjustment based on subjective perception and expectations honed by the reality of others. Conflict and the resulting balance form a structure of expectations that enables different views of injustice and different classes to live together.

In time these expectations may become incongruent with the underlying balance; a person may develop new reference groups, have new experiences, be the object of an ideological campaign ("workers are oppressed"). The sense of injustice may change such that the previous class balance (between workers and management in a factory) no longer reflects the parties' interests, or the underlying capabilities or wills of the parties may alter (bureaucratic dissension may weaken governmental control over dissidents). Then a trigger, such as an event provoking a rearoused or newly inflamed sense of injustice may provoke a turn of the conflict helix, a new balancing of powers and injustices, of classes.

At the *ontological and empirical levels* the nature of the psychological field and the conflict helix seems to answer the question, What is social justice? Just wants and injustice vectors vary considerably among people. Such interests and feelings are diverse, multidimensional, and *personal*. Moreover, the amount willingly sacrificed to satisfy just wants or to right a sense of injustice varies across individuals. People have different expectations, capabilities, interests, and wills. And the overriding superordinate goal, self-esteem, is intrinsic to the individual.

Then how, apparently, do we determine what is just? How do we balance different views of what is just? Given the diversity of human beings, this question can only imply two alternatives: we force our view of social justice on someone else (say, through governmental coercion), or people settle for themselves and among themselves their own balance. If the conflict helix as a field process operates at all levels without the imposition of an antifield on it, the diverse views of social justice will compromise and balance in terms of interests, capabilities, and wills. This seems to argue for the maximum freedom, for a precondition of the conflict helix is that each is free to pursue his just wants and to square his sense of injustice against others. The precondition of social justice is therefore freedom. Or, so it seems.

But this is a factual conclusion about an ethical question, which is not logically possible. Facts can be heuristic, they can provide some guidelines to thought, but they cannot make the argument themselves. To fully and logically answer the question we must consider the nature of ethics and then the ethical nature of social justice. Ultimately, we will have to use ethical arguments to determine what is socially just. And this I will do in the concluding volume of this series, *Vol. 5: The Just Peace*. There we will find that at the level of ethics we arrive at a conclusion similar to that we found ontologically and empirically: as a matter of ethics, social justice is the maximization of the freedom of individuals to choose the principles that govern them, even if they choose to be unfree.

Unrest

The general condition of the community in which milling is both frequent and widespread and in which rumour is recurrent is the crucible in which the more highly organized forms of collective behaviour develop. This condition, known as social unrest, can lead to outbursts of violence. The American urban black uprisings of the 1960s were preceded and accompanied by social unrest in the form of a rise in tensions in black communities throughout the country; the Russian Revolution was preceded by several years of constant unrest and turmoil, involving random assassinations, strikes, and riots.

There are several distinguishing characteristics to social unrest. First, there is a general impairment of collective life routines. People find it difficult to concentrate on their work or even to adhere to rules in playing games. Any occasion to abandon routines is welcomed. Second, people are hyperreactive. The magnitude of the response is out of proportion to the usual meaning of any stimulating incident. A small police provocation elicits a major outcry of police brutality; a trivial success is the occasion for large-scale celebration. Milling and rumour abound because incidents that would normally pass with little notice become occasions for both. Third, social unrest is marked by contagiousness. When restlessness is strictly individual, one person's restlessness merely annoys another. But when restlessness becomes a shared experience, people are highly suggestible to one another. Questioning and exploring alternative courses of action are reduced to a minimum. Fourth, social unrest is not specific with respect to grievances or activities. When there is social unrest in a school, students complain of both restrictions on their behaviour and the lack of clearly defined rules; they find fault both with school administrators and with their fellow students. Finally, social unrest is perhaps the most volatile of collective states. Unlike rumour or milling, it does not remain focused on an issue or problem. Unlike crowd behaviour or fads, it has not yet been channelled into one main direction. Although social unrest may eventually die down without any serious aftermath, it is a condition in which people can be easily aroused.

Adjustment and Maladjustment

In psychology, the Behavioural process by which humans and other animals maintain an equilibrium among their various needs or between their needs and the obstacles of their environments. A sequence of adjustment begins when a need is felt and ends when it is satisfied. Hungry people, for example, are stimulated by their physiological state to seek food. When they eat, they reduce the stimulating condition that impelled them to activity, and they are thereby adjusted to this particular need.

In general, the adjustment process involves four parts: (1) a need or motive in the form of a strong persistent stimulus, (2) the thwarting or nonfulfillment of this need, (3) varied activity, or exploratory behaviour accompanied by problem solving, and (4) some response that removes or at least reduces the initiating stimulus and completes the adjustment. Social and cultural adjustments are similar to physiological adjustments. People strive to be comfortable in their surroundings and to have their psychological needs (such as love or affirmation) met through the social networks they inhabit. When needs arise, especially in new or changed surroundings, they impel interpersonal activity meant to satisfy those needs. In this way, people increase their familiarity and comfort with their environments, and they come to expect that their needs will be met in the future through their social networks. Ongoing difficulties in social and cultural adjustment may be accompanied by anxiety or depression.

Causes of Maladjustment

The condition of being unable to adapt properly to your environment with resulting emotional instability.

1. Faulty or inadequate adjustment.
2. Inability to adjust to the demands of interpersonal relationships and the stresses of daily living.

Defence Mechanism

In Freudian psychoanalytic theory, **defence mechanisms** or **defense mechanisms** (see-ce/-se) are psychological strategies brought into play by various entities to cope with reality and to maintain self-image. Healthy persons normally use different defences throughout life. An ego defence mechanism becomes pathological only when its persistent use leads to maladaptive behaviour such that the physical and/or mental health of the individual is adversely affected. The purpose of the Ego Defence Mechanisms is to protect the mind/self/ego from anxiety, social sanctions or to provide a refuge from a situation with which one cannot currently cope.

They are more accurately referred to as ego defence mechanisms, and can thus be categorized as occurring when the id impulses are in conflict with each other, when the id impulses conflict with super-ego values and beliefs, and when an external threat is posed to the ego.

The term "defence mechanism" is often thought to refer to a definitive singular term for personality traits which arise due to loss or traumatic experiences, but more accurately refers to several types of reactions which were identified during and after daughter Anna Freud's time.

Mental Illness

A **mental disorder** or **mental illness** is a psychological or Behavioural pattern that occurs in an individual and is thought to cause distress or disability that is not expected as part of normal development or culture. The recognition and understanding of mental disorders has changed over time and across cultures. Definitions, assessments, and classifications of mental disorders can vary, but guideline criteria listed in the ICD, DSM and other manuals are widely accepted by mental health professionals. Categories of diagnoses in these schemes may include dissociative disorders, mood disorders, anxiety disorders, psychotic disorders, eating disorders, developmental disorders, personality disorders, and many other categories. In many cases there is no single accepted or consistent cause of mental disorders, although they are often explained in terms of a diathesis-stress model and biopsychosocial model. Mental disorders have been found to be common, with over a third of people in most countries reporting sufficient criteria at some point in their life. Services for mental disorders may be based in hospitals or in the community. Mental health professionals diagnose individuals using different methodologies, often relying on case history and interview. Psychotherapy and psychiatric medication are two major treatment options, as well as supportive interventions and self-help. Treatment may be involuntary where legislation allows. Several movements campaign for changes to services and attitudes.

Juvenile Delinquency

Juvenile delinquency refers to criminal acts performed by juveniles. Most legal systems prescribe specific procedures for dealing with juveniles, such as juvenile detention centers. There are a multitude of different theories on the causes of crime, most if not all of which can be applied to the causes of youth crime. Youth crime is an aspect of crime which receives great attention from the news media and politicians. Crime committed by young people has risen since the mid-twentieth century, as has most types of crime.

The level and types of youth crime can be used by commentators as an indicator of the general state of morality and law and order in a country, and consequently youth crime can be the source of 'moral panics' Theories on the causes of youth crime can be viewed as particularly important within criminology.

This is firstly because crime is committed disproportionately by those aged between fifteen and twenty-five. Secondly, by definition any theories on the causes of crime will focus on youth crime, as adult criminals will have likely started offending when they were young. A Juvenile Delinquent is one who repeatedly commits crime, however these juvenile delinquents could most likely have mental disorders/Behavioural issues such as schizophrenia, post traumatic stress disorder or bipolar disorder.

Theoretical Perspectives on Juvenile Delinquency

Rational Choice Theory

Classical criminology stresses that causes of crime lie within the individual offender, rather than in their external environment. For classicists, offenders are motivated by rational self-interest, and the importance of free will and personal responsibility is emphasised.

Rational choice theory is the clearest example of this approach. It states that people weigh the pros and cons of committing a crime, and offend when the former outweigh the latter. A central deficiency of rational choice theory is that while it may explain when and where people commit crime, it can't explain very well why people choose to commit crimes in the first place.

Neither can it explain differences between individuals and groups in their propensity to commit crimes. James Q. Wilson said the conscience and self-control of a potential young offender must be taken into account, and that these attributes are formed by parental and societal conditioning. Rational choice does not explain why crime should be committed disproportionately by young people, males, city dwellers, and the poor. (Walklate: 2003 p.2)

It also ignores the influence a young choice theory does not take into account the proven correlations between certain social circumstances and individuals' personalities, and the propensity to commit crime.

Social Disorganization Theory

Current positivist approaches generally focus on the Culture, which would produce the breakdown of family relationships and community, competing values, and increasing Individualism.

Studies also show only 16 in every 100 kids will do something bad opposed to adult 26 in 100 will do something bad or illegal.

Strain Theory

Strain Theory is associated mainly with the work of Robert Merton. He felt that there are institutionalized paths to success in society. Strain theory holds that crime is caused by the difficulty those in poverty have in achieving socially valued goals by legitimate means.

As those with, for instance, poor educational attainment have difficulty achieving wealth and status by securing well paid employment, they are more likely to use criminal means to obtain these goals. Merton's suggests five adaptations to this dilemma:

1. *Innovation*: individuals who accept socially approved goals, but not necessarily the socially approved means.
2. *Retreatism*: those who reject socially approved goals and the means for acquiring them.
3. *Ritualism*: those who buy into a system of socially approved means, but lose sight of the goals. Merton believed that drug users are in this category.
4. *Conformity*: those who conform to the system's means and goals.

5. *Rebellion*: people who negate socially approved goals and means by creating a new system of acceptable goals and means.

A difficulty with strain theory is that it does not explore why children of low-income families would have poor educational attainment in the first place. More importantly is the fact that much youth crime does not have an economic motivation. Strain theory fails to explain violent crime, the type of youth crime which causes most anxiety to the public.

Subcultural Theory

Related to strain theory is subcultural theory. The inability of youths to achieve socially valued status and goals results in groups of young people forming deviant or delinquent subcultures, which have their own values and norms. (Eadie & Morley: 2003 p.552) Within these groups criminal behaviour may actually be valued, and increase a youth's status. (Walklate: 2003 p.22)

The notion of delinquent subcultures is relevant for crimes that are not economically motivated. Male gang members could be argued to have their own values, such as respect for fighting ability and daring. However it is not clear how different this makes them from 'ordinary' non-lawbreaking young men. Furthermore there is no explanation of why people unable to achieve socially valued goals should necessarily choose criminal substitutes. Subcultural theories have been criticised for making too sharp a distinction between what is deviant and what is 'normal'. (Brown: 1998 p.23) There are also doubts about whether young people consciously reject mainstream values. (Brown: 1998 p.23)

Differential Association

The theory of Differential association also deals with young people in a group context, and looks at how peer pressure and the existence of gangs could lead them into crime. It suggests young people are motivated to commit crimes by delinquent peers, and learn criminal skills from them. The diminished influence of peers after men marry has also been cited as a factor in desisting from offending. There is strong evidence that young people with criminal friends are more likely to commit crimes themselves.

However it may be the case that offenders prefer to associate with one another, rather than delinquent peers causing someone to start offending. Furthermore there is the question of how the delinquent peer group became delinquent initially.

Labelling Theory

Labelling theory states that once young people have been libelled as criminal they are more likely to offend. (Eadie & Morley: 2003 p.552)

The idea is that once labelled as deviant a young person may accept that role, and be more likely to associate with others who have been similarly labelled. (Eadie & Morley: 2003 p.552)

Labelling theorists say that male children from poor families are more likely to be labelled deviant, and that this may partially explain why there are more lower-class young male offenders. (Walklate: 2003 p. 24)

Juvenile Delinquency as a Male Phenomenon

Youth crime is disproportionately committed by young men. Feminist theorists and others have examined why this is the case. (Eadie & Morley: 2003 p.553) One suggestion is that ideas of masculinity may make young men more likely to offend. Being tough, powerful, aggressive, daring and competitive may be a way of young men expressing their masculinity. (Brown: 1998 p.109) Acting out these ideals may make young men more likely to engage in antisocial and criminal behaviour. (Walklate: 2003 p. 83)

Alternatively, rather than young men acting as they do because of societal pressure to conform to masculine ideals; young men may actually be naturally more aggressive, daring etc. As well as biological or psychological factors, the way young men are treated by their parents may make them more susceptible to offending. (Walklate: 2003 p. 35) According to a study led by Florida State University criminologist Kevin M.

Beaver, adolescent males who possess a certain type of variation in a specific gene are more likely to flock to delinquent peers. The study, which appears in the September 2008 issue of the Journal of Genetic Psychology, is the first to establish a statistically significant association between an affinity for antisocial peer groups and a particular variation (called the 10-repeat allele) of the dopamine transporter gene (DAT1).

Promotion of Mental Health of Students and Teachers

Teachers are among the most important influences in the lives of school-aged children, yet relatively little emphasis has been placed on examining the potential role general academic teachers may play in facilitating adolescent health promotion efforts, according to a study conducted by researchers at Columbia University's Mailman School of Public Health and published in the *Journal of School Health*. The study results indicate that teachers provide valuable information to school personnel about what health issues are important to adolescents, in particular, because they hear feedback from adolescents on a daily basis.

"We found that teachers agreed that schools were an important venue for discussing and providing health messages," says Alwyn T. Cohall, MD, associate professor of clinical Sociomedical Sciences, director of the Harlem Health Promotion Centre, and lead author. "However, they expressed concern about their ability to handle mental health, Behavioural health, and reproductive health problems, and desire additional staff development workshops to address these needs."

More than half (52%) of those surveyed overheard student discussions about health once a week or more in classrooms, hallways, cafeterias, and playgrounds. Seventy percent of teachers stated they were actively approached by students one to three times per semester or more with personal problems or health concerns.

"Our study shows that relying solely on certified health education teachers to impart health messages and facilitate referrals for services would appear rather limiting given these contextual realities," noted Dr. Cohall.

While approximately 90% of U.S. school districts require health education in public schools, relatively little emphasis has been placed on examining the role that non-health teachers play in facilitating adolescent health promotion efforts. Yet, teachers are among the most important influences in the lives of school-aged children ages six to 18.

"It is conceivable that almost all teachers have opportunities, both formal and informal, to influence adolescent health behaviour. However, to our knowledge, there have been few studies that examine the extent to which general academic teachers are involved in interactions with students about health," observed Dr. Cohall.

The survey was conducted among academic teachers and administrators working in four schools in the Northern Manhattan community of New York City. These schools had a cumulative enrolment of approximately 4,600 students, and an active school-based health clinic on site, providing a wide range of free physical and mental health services to students during school hours, including primary and reproductive healthcare.

The teachers surveyed believe that schools are an appropriate place for discussion and dissemination of health information. Yet, the data indicates that fewer than 20% of the teachers had provided formal classroom material on a health topic such as nutrition (19.8%), tobacco, drugs or alcohol (19.0%), reproductive health (17.2%), mental health (15%); less than 8% planned to provide such material in the future.

In general, teachers described themselves as being reasonably comfortable addressing many of these problems. They were less comfortable discussing problems at home, emotional or mental health, and medical problems or illness. Sixty-three percent of teachers surveyed indicated they had referred a student to the school-based clinic, suggesting that teachers play an important role in facilitating care for youth.

More than three quarters of teachers were interested in receiving staff development on problems with peers (77.5%) and emotional or mental health (77.3%). The other two areas where more than half of the teachers were interested in receiving staff development were problems at home and reproductive health issues related to sex, pregnancy, and sexually transmitted infections.

Teachers were approached by students regardless of race/ethnicity. The implied impression of teachers as approachable, credible sources of information, regardless of race/ethnicity, has important implications. For example, research has consistently shown that students who feel connected to their schools are less likely to engage in risky behaviour.

"Our findings suggest the need for closer and more consistent interactions between school-based clinic staff and school personnel throughout the year, and points out the need for further research to develop cost-effective and time-efficient strategies to enhance the health literacy of all school personnel," said Dr. Cohall.

Unit-X

Guidance and Counselling

Nature, Types and Need of Guidance and Counselling—Educational, Vocational and Personal

Guidance is assistance given to an individual to help him, to adjust to himself, to others and to his own peculiar environment. Guidance helps him to understand himself. It helps him in his acquaintance with the things and the world around him. Finally, it helps the person to seek harmony between his personal needs and ambitions with peculiarities of his own environment. In this way, guidance can be described as a process of assisting an individual with his adjustment problems. Thus, according to Jones, "Guidance is the help given by one person to another in making choices and adjustments and in solving problems". While Skinner says "Guidance is a process of helping young persons learns to adjust to self, to others, and to circumstances".

Guidance aims to prepare an individual for his future life. It helps him to acquire essential skills, abilities and capacities for the tasks to be accomplished in future. It also helps the individual in selecting a proper future profession and role in the society and enables him to play his role successfully. Guidance has personal and social significance. It aims to help an individual in the process of his adjustment with himself and his environment. It helps him to develop his strengths and abilities, to achieve utmost personal and social efficiency. It also aims to stop wastage of human power and physical resources by helping the individuals to find their place in society.

Thus, we can say that **GUIDANCE** is the process of helping an individual to help himself and to develop his potentialities to the fullest by utilizing the maximum opportunities provided by the environment.

Guidance and Counselling

On the other hand, COUNSELLING is the service offered to the individual, who is undergoing a problem and needs professional help to overcome it. The problem keeps him disturbed, high strung, under tension and unless solved, his development is hampered or stunted. Counselling therefore, is a more specialized service requiring training in personality development and handling exceptional groups of individuals. For example, individuals suffering from sensory handicaps like, visually handicapped, deaf and mute, speech disorders, or from physical handicaps like malfunctioning of glands or vital organs; orthopaedically handicapped; personal-social handicaps like, neurotics, psychotics, depressed isolates or from intellectual retardation or exceptionally high talent and so on. In other words, when the development is not normal because of certain handicaps, the individual needs help to be able to adjust to the environmental pressures and learn to overcome his handicaps or at least accept them squarely.

COUNSELLING services are therefore, required for individuals having developmental problems, because of the handicap they suffer in any area of growth like, physical, mental, moral, social and emotional, either because of hereditary factors or environmental conditions.

Counselling therefore is offered to only those individuals who are under serious problem and need professional help to overcome it, while guidance is needed by all at any time.

Both guidance and counselling assist the individual to know about himself, to adjust himself, with others and the environment and thus lead the individual to become a WHOLESOME PERSON.

Philosophy of Guidance

Guidance is universal and the basic principles of the philosophy of guidance are common to all countries with a slight modification to suit the locally accepted beliefs and the specific guidance services offered. The eight principles of the philosophy of guidance are:

1. The dignity of the individual is supreme.
2. Each individual is unique. He or she is different from every other individual.
3. The primary concern of guidance is the individual in his own social setting. The main aim being to help him to become a wholesome person and to gain fullest satisfaction in his life.
4. The attitudes and personal perceptions of the individual are the bases on which he acts.
5. The individual generally acts to enhance his perceived self.
6. The individual has the innate ability to learn and can be helped to make choices that will lead to self-direction, and make him consistent with the social environment.
7. The individual needs a continuous guidance process from early childhood through adulthood.
8. Each individual may, at times, need the information and personalized assistance best given by competent professional personnel.

The Goals to Achieve in Guidance

At present, Guidance has taken an unprecedented lead over all the other helping professions, for it empowers an individual to charter his life successfully, inspite of all odds.

The main goals are:

1. Exploring-self: The basic aim is to help an individual increase his understanding and acceptance of self; his physical development, his intelligence, aptitudes, interest, personality traits, attitudes and values, his achievements in scholastic and other spheres, his aspirations and life-style preferences and above all his here-and-now needs which keep him highly motivated to behave positively *or otherwise.*

2. Determining Values: The second aim is to help an individual recognize the importance of values, explore different sets of values, determine personal values and examine them in relation to the norms of society and their importance in planning for success in life.
3. Setting Goals: This aim is to help an individual set goal for him self and relate these to the values determined by him so that he recognizes the importance of long-range planning.
4. Explore the World of Work: The aim here is to help the individual explore the World of Work in relation to his self-exploration, his value system and goals that he has set for himself to achieve success in life.
5. Improving Efficiency: The individual is helped to learn about factors which contribute to increase effectiveness and efficiency and to improve his study habits.
6. Building Relationship: The aim is to help the individual to be aware of his relationship with others and to note that it is a reflection of his own feelings about himself.
7. Accepting responsibility for the future: The individual is helped to develop skill in social and personal forecasting, acquire attitudes and skills necessary for mastering the future.

To sum up, guidance empowers him to be an integrated individual, actualizing his potential to the fullest.

What are the Main Types of Counselling?

Individual Counselling

A counsellor can meet with you on a one-to-one basis, with you and your partner or with members of your family, to talk through issues that are concerning you.

Group Therapy

A counsellor leads the discussion for a group of people (with or without similar issues of concern) who get together on a regular basis to share their experiences or concerns.

Online and Telephone Counselling

Working with a counsellor online, by telephone, by Email, chat-room or instant messaging is certainly not as good as face-to-face counselling but can be very effective when there are long distances involved. This is especially relevant in India, USA, UK & France.

Self-help Groups

People who are experiencing similar problems, such as loss and grief, trauma, divorce and illness, meet to discuss common issues and problems (with or without a counsellor to lead the discussion).

Vocational Guidance Education in the Curriculum

The national curriculum provides for **educational** and **vocational guidance** activities to be offered in primary and secondary education, through a distinct subject named **Counselling** and **Guidance**. This subject is included in the common core curriculum for all of compulsory education, covering mainly **educational** aspects in primary education, and both **educational** and **vocational** aspects in secondary education.

The framework objectives defined for **Counselling** and **Guidance** are the following:

- development of a positive attitude towards oneself as unique and valuable person;
- development of knowledge, skills and attitudes related to interpersonal aspects;
- development of skills necessary to use various types of information in the learning process;
- development of skills necessary in career exploration and planning;
- practice of management skills related to a quality lifestyle.

Traineeships within the Framework of the Curriculum

Schools are encouraged to establish partnerships with companies and other institutions at local level in order to contribute to the development of local communities and to familiarise pupils with the professional world.

After the first four years of general lower secondary education *(gimnaziu)*, pupils must continue with two more years of lower secondary education in another institution. Those attending either the technological branch of secondary school *(Liceu)* or the Arts and Trades School participate – for a period of 3 weeks for the former and 10 weeks for the latter – in traineeships and work placements in public or private companies. These activities are based on the specific syllabi approved by the Ministry of Education, Research and Youth.

Educational, Vocational Counsellor

Counsel students regarding educational issues such as course and program selection, class scheduling, school adjustment, truancy, study habits, and career planning. Counsel individuals to help them understand and overcome personal, social, or Behavioural problems affecting their educational or vocational situations. Maintain accurate and complete student records as required by laws, district policies, and administrative regulations. Confer with parents or guardians, teachers, other Counsellors, and administrators to resolve students' Behavioural, academic, and other problems. Provide crisis intervention to students when difficult situations occur at schools.

Identify cases involving domestic abuse or other family problems affecting students' development. Meet with parents and guardians to discuss their children's progress, and to determine their priorities for their children and their resource needs. Prepare students for later educational experiences by encouraging them to explore learning opportunities and to persevere with challenging tasks. Encourage students and/or parents to seek additional assistance from mental health professionals when necessary. Observe and evaluate students' performance, behaviour, social development, and physical health. Enforce all administration policies and rules governing students. Meet with other professionals to discuss individual students' needs and progress.

Provide students with information on such topics as college degree programs and admission requirements, financial aid opportunities, trade and technical schools, and apprenticeship programs. Evaluate individuals' abilities, interests, and personality characteristics using tests, records, interviews, and professional sources. Collaborate with teachers and administrators in the development, evaluation, and revision of school programs. Teach classes and present self-help or information sessions on subjects related to education and career planning. Establish and enforce Behavioural rules and procedures to maintain order among students. Conduct follow-up interviews with counselees to determine if their needs have been met. Attend professional meetings, educational conferences, and teacher training workshops, in order to maintain and improve professional competence. Prepare reports on students and activities as required by administration.

Plan and conduct orientation programs and group conferences to promote the adjustment of individuals to new life experiences such as starting college. Assess needs for assistance such as rehabilitation, financial aid, or additional vocational training, and refer clients to the appropriate services. Instruct individuals in career development techniques such as job search and application strategies, resume writing, and interview skills. Address community groups, faculty, and staff members to explain available counselling services. Attend staff meetings, and serve on committees as required. Compile and study occupational, educational, and economic information to assist counselees in determining and carrying out vocational and educational objectives.

Provide information for teachers and staff members involved in helping students or graduates identify and pursue employment opportunities. Review transcripts to ensure that students meet graduation or college entrance requirements, and write letters of recommendation. Refer students to degree programs based on interests, aptitudes, or educational assessments. Provide special services such as alcohol and drug prevention programs, and classes that teach students to handle conflicts without resorting to violence. Provide disabled students with assistive devices, supportive technology, and assistance accessing facilities such as restrooms.

Observe children during classroom and play activities to gain additional information about them. Interview clients to obtain information about employment history, educational background, and career goals, and to identify barriers to employment. Establish and supervise peer counselling and peer tutoring programs. Plan and promote career and employment-related programs such as work-experience programs. Refer qualified counselees to employers or employment services for job placement. Sponsor extracurricular activities such as clubs, student organizations, and academic contests. Perform administrative duties such as hall and cafeteria monitoring, and bus loading and unloading. Provide information to businesses regarding human resource and employment issues.

Identification of Children with Counselling Needs

Counselling concerns of highly able students may reflect characteristics associated with giftedness. Yet school counsellor A school counsellor is a counsellor and educator who works in schools, and have historically been referred to as "guidance Counsellors" or "educational Counsellors," although "Professional School Counsellor" is now the preferred term training programs give scant attention to this phenomenon and to the social and emotional development of these students. School Counsellors therefore may be unaware of and unequipped Adj. 1. unequipped-without necessary physical or intellectual equipment; "guerrillas unequipped for a pitched battle"; "unequipped for jobs in a modern technological society" to respond to these concerns. Referencing scholarly literature related to giftedness as both asset and burden, the author explores school counsellors' potential roles in responding to the needs of gifted students.

According to according to *prep.*

1. As stated or indicated by; on the authority of: according to historians.

2. In keeping with: according to instructions.
3. a recent unpublished study (Peterson, 2005) of school counselling graduate programs (53% response rate) accredited recognition by an appropriate authority that the performance of a particular institution has satisfied a prestated set of criteria.

Accredited Herds

Cattle herds which have achieved a low level of reactors to, e.g. by the Council for Accreditation of Counselling and Related Educational Programs, preparatory curricula give little or no attention to the unique developmental concerns and counselling issues related to high ability. Only 62% of programs gave any attention at all in their entire preparatory program, and 47% devoted three or fewer contact hours. Such little emphasis on the overlay:

(1) A preprinted, precut form placed over a screen, key or tablet for identification purposes.

(2) A program segment called into memory when required of characteristics associated with giftedness on social and emotional development, on both assets and burdens of high capability, and on the need for differential counselling responses suggests that school Counsellors may not understand or respond appropriately to counselling concerns of those students. Furthermore, like other educators who may be unaware of complex affective /af·fec·tive/ (ah-fek´tiv) pertaining to affect.

Counselling Issues

Curricula, conceptions of intelligence, measurement, and characteristics of giftedness have received considerable focus in research related to education of gifted students. Neihart, Reis, Robinson, and Moon's (2002) compilation of research related to social and emotional development of gifted individuals attended to acceleration, attributions, gender differences, cultural differences, creativity, learning disabilities, deficits in attention, motivation, career development, underachievement, and asynchronous Refers to events that are not synchronized, or coordinated, in time. The following are considered asynchronous operations. The interval between transmitting A and B is not the same as between B and C. The ability to initiate a transmission at either end development (e.g., cognitive development outpacing social and emotional development, Silverman, 1997). Findings in these areas have implications for social and emotional development, of course.

However, Moon (2003) noted the heavy emphasis in the field on achievement outcomes, to the neglect of "other important outcomes, such as happiness, well-being, and life satisfaction" and "helping students develop self-awareness and skills in decision making and self-regulation" (p. 16). Actually, school Counsellors, gifted-education and classroom teachers (Peterson, 2003), and university-based counselling centers serving gifted youth (Colangelo & Assouline, 2000) can provide appropriate services, and parent groups (Webb & DeVries, 1993) can indirectly offer support. Private and agency Counsellors (Mahoney, 1997; Mendaglio, 2005) also can provide services for gifted individuals that are as tailored to individual needs and developmental levels as are services for others. In this case, approaches are selected with exceptional ability and related characteristics and concerns in mind. Yet counselling issues and approaches generally have received little attention in the scholarly literature related to giftedness (Reis & Moon, 2002). Characteristics associated with high capability may contribute to counselling needs regardless of culture or socioeconomic status socioeconomic status, *n* the position of an individual on a socio-economic scale that measures such factors as education, income, type of occupation, place of residence, and in some populations, ethnicity and religion..

Among several issues related to educating and counselling gifted students, it is important for school Counsellors to be aware of identification practices, because problems inherent in these may be related to counselling concerns. Large numbers of bright, sensitive, creative, and insightful children and adolescents, representing the full range of cultural and socioeconomic contexts, may not be identified for programs for gifted and talented students (Birely & Genshaft, 1991; Ford, 1996). Yet these students might especially benefit from having their gifts affirmed and nurtured through participation in a program (Peterson, 1997).

A standardized test A **standardized test** is a test administered and scored in a standard manner. The tests are designed in such a way that the "questions, conditions for administering, scoring procedures, and interpretations are consistent" often serves as the gateway to participation (Coleman, Gallagher, & Foster, 1994). However, classroom teachers may be asked to refer students for evaluation whose scores on the standardized tests used for initial screening did not qualify them. When teachers consider potential nominees, cultural factors may then play a role, because cultural values have an impact on classroom behaviour, teacher-student relationships, students' fit in the school environment, and identification of students for special programs (Peterson, 1999). In one ethnographic eth·nog·ra·phy *n.*

Work Ethic

Noun

A belief in the moral value of work, social status, and social skills) might preclude identification of children from cultures that do not value verbal assertiveness and "standing out," as well as students with low English proficiency, behaviour problems, low socioeconomic status, and poor social skills.

Limiting participation to students who achieve well on group tests and in the classroom also leaves out highly able students whose difficult life circumstances, skeptical attitudes about school, lack of parental support (Peterson, 1997), learning and physical disabilities (Olenchak & Reis, 2002), depression (Jackson, 1998), behaviour problems (Neihart, 2002a), and even temporary or chronic illness might preclude optimal test performance. Regardless of whether their circumstances may change during or after the school years, opportunities for crucial affirmation and support are lost. Teachers and even school Counsellors may not recognize their ability, even if behaviour problems and emotional distress emotional distress n. an increasingly popular basis for a claim of damages in lawsuits for injury due to the negligence or intentional acts of another.

Originally damages for emotional distress were only awardable in conjunction with damages for actual physical harm bring these students to their attention.

Sensitivity, intensity, drivenness (Lovecky, 1992), and developmental asynchrony asynchrony /asyn·chro·ny/

1. lack of synchronism; disturbance of coordination.
2. occurrence at distinct times of events normally synchronous; disturbance of coordination. asynchronous (Silverman, 1997), rather than disability or pathology or a "bad attitude," may actually be at the root of behaviour problems. In general, school Counsellors and other mental health professionals may not recognize that these may be related to giftedness (Webb et al., 2005). Such misinterpretation of behaviours can lead to emotional distress (Moon, 2003), and stress can contribute to depression and anxiety. Some troubled gifted students may self-medicate with substances (Peterson, 1998).

In summary, school Counsellors should be aware tnat intellectually gifted and otherwise highly talented nonmainstream students may not be identified either by standardized tests or by teacher nominations. It is important that school Counsellors be alert to abilities that become evident through guidance-related contact or examination of school records over time. Gifted students may be at risk for poor outcomes for a variety of reasons (Peterson, 1997, 2002), and giftedness in itself can be a risk factor. Lack of affirmation from self and others regarding high capability may actually be a presenting issue and can be addressed in counselling.

Counselling Techniques

Introduction

You need many years of practice and usually a qualification to become an accomplished counsellor. However, anyone, regardless of qualifications and training can become a more effective helper by learning to apply the basic techniques of counselling. These are as follows:

Getting the Environment Right

If you feel that it is safe to do so, create a space to talk which is private and quiet and where you know you will be free from interruptions (always seek the advice of a colleague about the safety and appropriateness of this action). Where possible, make sure the seating is comfortable and make sure that there is appropriate heating and ventilation.

Get the message across that you have time to attend to the issue that you want to address. Get the message across that the conversation is private and that you will not be passing on what the child/young person says to any third party*.

* You have to also make it clear that if the child/young person gives you information that suggests that they or others are in danger (for example a disclosure of abuse or threat of self-harm) you cannot keep this confidential. *Make sure that you are fully aware of your organisation's child protection policies.*

Getting the Listening Right

One way of encouraging a child or young person to talk is to make sure that they know you are listening. You can do this by just being attentive and by showing with your body language that you are listening. Sometimes this will be by facing the child and making good eye contact. Sometimes sitting side by side (for example during a journey) will be less threatening. Try not to interrupt when the child/young person is talking. By occasionally nodding or quietly saying "yes" or "aha" the child/young person should be encouraged to open up. Reporting back to the child a short summary of what they have just said and asking them if you have got it right is another way of doing this. Make sure you look and sound calm, unhurried and caring.

Asking the Right Questions

Try to ask more open questions than closed questions.

An open question is one which cannot be answered with yes or no and which encourages a more detailed answer, for example:

- *"What are your feelings about this?"*
- *"What are the advantages of doing things the way you have suggested?"*
- *"What are the disadvantages?"*

Avoid closed questions such as:

- *"Are you sad?"*
- *"Are you looking forward to the school holidays?"*

Another disadvantage of closed questioning is that the desired answer might be implied within the question and you might inadvertently steer the child/young person to give an answer that they wouldn't otherwise have given. An example of this would be:

"Are you going to stop speaking to that boy who has been upsetting you?"

The implied expected answer here is quite clearly *"yes"*.

Being Affirming

To encourage the flow of conversation it is important that you show respect by taking an accepting attitude. The message you are trying to get across is "I have respect for your opinions and your view of the world at this present time". This is not the same as saying that you agree with the child's opinions or actions and it is okay for you to make it clear that your opinions and moral view are different, as long as this is done in a respectful way.

"[child] seemed to really bond with [worker]-she spoke to him as if he was a person rather than focusing on his behaviour. If he had done well she praised him, which he responds to"

Career

Limiting the Advice

Try to limit the direct advice that you give during your conversation. This is more important for older than for younger children who clearly need more guidance. This is especially the case at the beginning of a piece of problem-solving conversation. For example, it is usually better to start with "What do you think is the best thing for you to do next?" than to say, "What you should do next is..."

How to make it Work?

- Do not turn your conversation into an interrogation. However good you are at counselling some children/ young people will not be ready to talk to you or want to talk to you. This does not mean that you have failed. It might be that they will talk later or that they will talk to a colleague of yours who they know better or a colleague of the opposite sex.
- Make sure that you recognise when you are getting out of your depth. If your conversation with a child/young person uncovers clear evidence of abuse or serious mental distress/ill health, seek immediate advice from your local mental health specialist team.
- After your conversation with a child/young person make sure that you take time out to reflect with a colleague or supervisor about the interaction that you have had.

Individual and Group Techniques

A Comparative Analysis of the Two Methods of Therapy

Counselling is a process whereby the relationship and communication provided allows development of understanding of one's self, explore possibilities, and initiate change. It is motivated by care and concern for the well-being of the recipient, and aim at bringing about Behavioural change, problem-solving, personal growth and development when properly implemented.

Advantages of Individual Counselling

The advantages of an individual counselling as opposed to group counselling are multiple:

- First, it allows the counsellor to work in isolated issues.
- Second, the counsellor caters only to one client.
- Third, the information gathered is easier for the counsellor to figure out and to be able to apply which treatment approach is most useful to the client and target behaviour that needs improvement.

- The client's thoughts and behaviours may not be distorted compared with group counselling as several pattern of thoughts and behaviours from other group members in making choices and decision making.
- The client has the power to change his life for the better based on the choices he make.
- In addition to this, he can control his behaviour and that the level of commitment and how hard he is willing to work will dictate how successful he will be in developing new behaviours that clearly communicate his needs in accordance with William Glasser's Reality Therapy.

Disadvantages of Individual Therapy

- The disadvantages of an individual therapy include the client's choice is solely from him.
- The client may not able to generate ideas from other members' pattern of thoughts and behaviours just like in a group setting especially if others have similar issues and experiences which could help him make better choices and decision making.

Group counselling is more in consonance with the Control Theory, later named Choice Theory, forwarded by William Glasser. This theory states that a person's behaviour is inspired by what that person wants or needs at that particular time, not on an outside stimulus.

That all living creatures control their behaviour to fulfil their need for satisfaction in one or more of these five areas: survival, to belong and be loved by others, to have power and importance, freedom and independence, and to have fun. The most important need among the five is love and belongingness. Group counselling promotes this kind of feeling. Being connected to others is encouraged in group counselling.

Advantages of Group Counselling

- Group counselling is better than individual counselling when it comes to developing new behaviours that clearly communicate their needs and help in attaining fulfilment in the reality. Group therapy considers the key elements of what the group are looking for and what will make their life better, what the group will do to bring about what they want and how they are able to make alternative options and come up with common plan.

- Group counselling also provides members with the opportunities to learn with and from other people and to be able to understand own patterns of thoughts and behaviours, as well as those of others. Other people may see attitudes and behaviour patterns that are limiting and difficult to see in self.
- A group is an opportunity to receive genuine support, honest feedback, and useful alternatives from peers. It also enables members to experiment and work towards improved attitudes and ways of coping with stress. A group may also help individuals with relationship concerns and general difficulties in dealing with other people.

Humans are social creatures by nature and that our primary need is to love and belong. It is therefore essential that we have the capacity to develop and maintain relationships because it is through people that our other needs can be met.

Presenting problems are a result of poor, unfulfilling, or conflict-ridden relationships or the absence of relationships. William Glasser's Choice Theory is applicable in group counselling wherein the group may be able to make effective choices and take greater responsibility.

Disadvantages of Group Counselling

Group counselling has some disadvantages:

- too such as reflecting too many feelings and listening to far too many long stories;
- insufficient group member movement and involvement;
- not using creative techniques to get and hold the attention of the group members;
- not supporting techniques with theory and focusing the group sessions insufficiently.

Given the above advantages and disadvantages for individual or group format, it is up to the patient which one serves him or her best.

Guidance for the Children with Learning Difficulties, Under Achievers and Gifted

Parents are often worried when their child has learning problems in school. There are many reasons for school failure, but a common one is a specific learning disability. Children with learning disabilities usually have a normal range of intelligence. They try very hard to follow instructions, concentrate, and "be good" at home and in school. Yet, despite this effort, he or she is not mastering school tasks and falls behind. Learning disabilities affect at least 1 in 10 schoolchildren.

It is believed that learning disabilities are caused by a difficulty with the nervous system that affects receiving, processing, or communicating information. They may also run in families. Some children with learning disabilities are also hyperactive; unable to sit still, easily distracted, and have a short attention span.

Child and adolescent psychiatrists point out that learning disabilities are treatable. If not detected and treated early, however, they can have a tragic "snowballing" effect. For instance, a child who does not learn addition in elementary school cannot understand algebra in high school. The child, trying very hard to learn, becomes more and more frustrated, and develops emotional problems such as low self-esteem in the face of repeated failure. Some learning disabled children misbehave in school because they would rather be seen as "bad" than "stupid." Parents should be aware of the most frequent signals of learning disabilities, when a child:

- has difficulty understanding and following instructions.
- has trouble remembering what someone just told him or her.
- fails to master reading, spelling, writing, and/or math skills, and thus fails

- has difficulty distinguishing right from left; difficulty identifying words or a tendency to reverse letters, words, or numbers; (for example, confusing 25 with 52, "b" with "d," or "on" with "no").
- lacks coordination in walking, sports, or small activities such as holding a pencil or tying a shoelace.
- easily loses or misplaces homework, schoolbooks, or other items.
- cannot understand the concept of time; is confused by "yesterday, today, tomorrow."

Such problems deserve a comprehensive evaluation by an expert who can assess all of the different issues affecting the child. A child and adolescent psychiatrist can help coordinate the evaluation, and work with school professionals and others to have the evaluation and educational testing done to clarify if a learning disability exists.

This includes talking with the child and family, evaluating their situation, reviewing the educational testing, and consulting with the school.

The child and adolescent psychiatrist will then make recommendations on appropriate school placement, the need for special help such as special educational services or speech-language therapy and help parents assist their child in maximizing his or her learning potential.

Sometimes individual or family psychotherapy will be recommended. Medication may be prescribed for hyperactivity or distractibility. It is important to strengthen the child's self-confidence, so vital for healthy development, and also help parents and other family members better understand and cope with the realities of living with a child with learning disabilities.

Oppositional Behaviour as a Learning Disability: Guidance Pediatricians Can Offer Parents

Description

Counselling parents about noncompliance and disruptive behaviour.

"He won't listen!!"

Noncompliance and temper outbursts are among the most common of parental concerns. Most children will display some mild noncompliance and temper outbursts, but when the frequency and severity of these behaviours are beyond the norm the adverse impact on parent-child interactions and families can be dramatic and the long-term ramifications potentially significant.

Parents are often eager for a greater understanding of their child's difficulties; uncertain about the conflicting wisdom of myriad "self-help" books, mental health professionals, friends, and relatives; and unclear as to whether pharmacologic intervention would be helpful.

Your Explanation Guides Your Intervention

Conventional wisdom might lead us to believe that noncompliance and temper outbursts are the byproduct of inconsistent, non-contingent parenting, and would therefore lead us to dispense guidance aimed at helping parents to be more consistent and contingent.

Time-out from reinforcement (or other punishments) and contingency management programs (by which certain behaviours are targeted and closely monitored and children receive various reinforcers if Behavioural goals are met) are the familiar tools of such help.

While such strategies are generally supported by the research literature (Brestan & Eyberg, 1998), this same literature also clearly indicates that they do not benefit a substantial percentage of parents and children, especially over the long-term and especially as the intensity and severity of noncompliance and temper outbursts increases.

Researchers have recently shown that oppositional behaviour in children almost always occurs within the context of other comorbid conditions, including:

- executive dysfunction (as might be seen in ADHD);
- difficulties in social information processing;
- language processing impairments;

- difficulties in emotion regulation (as might be seen in children diagnosed with depression, bipolar disorder, or anxiety disorders);
- rigid, concrete, literal, black-and-white thinking (as might be seen in children with Asperger's disorder or non-verbal learning disability);
- sensory hyper-or hypo-sensitivity (Greene et al., 2002).

Oppositional defiant disorder (ODD)-the somewhat controversial label applied to children whose level of noncompliance and temper outbursts renders them "diagnosable"-rarely occurs outside the context of these comorbid conditions. Thus, how one interprets this overlap is important.

One interpretation has been offered by Greene and colleagues (Greene, 2001; Greene & Ablon, 2003; Greene, Ablon, & Goring, 2003), who have argued that each of these comorbid conditions has the potential to compromise a child's skills in several important cognitive domains: flexibility, frustration tolerance, and problem solving. From this perspective, oppositional behaviour is conceptualized as a developmental learning disability that results from a lag in the development of critical skills.

Naturally, if a child is lacking crucial cognitive skills, the goals of intervention are to understand the factors contributing to the skill-deficit and to teach the lacking skills. If so, then careful consideration must be given to how one goes about achieving this understanding, and whether commonly recommended behaviour management strategies actually teach lacking cognitive skills.

Teaching Cognitive Skills

The **Collaborative Problem Solving** (CPS) approach (Greene, 2001; Greene & Ablon, 2003; Greene et al., 2003) is a multi-faceted model of psychosocial treatment that specifically aims at teaching cognitive skills that are lacking in noncompliant and explosive children. It focuses on helping adults to effectively collaborate with children to resolve the issues that have been precipitating explosive outbursts. The CPS model delineates three common ways in which adults respond to problems or unmet expectations in their children. One mode of response-for ease of exposition, referred to as "Basket A"-involves the imposition of adult will. Another approach-referred to as "Basket C"-involves dropping or removing the expectation, at least temporarily. The third mode of responding-"Basket B"-involves engaging the child in a process of "collaborative problem solving" so as to resolve whatever issues or problems are precipitating explosive outbursts.

Basket A	Basket B	Basket C
Adult imposes will on child	Engage child in "Collaborative Problem Solving"	Temporarily remove expectation

Rather than helping adults become highly skilled at imposing their will (Basket A), the CPS model instead teaches and encourages adults to engage children in collaborative problem solving (Basket B).

Basket B serves several important functions.

1. Over time, Basket B helps adults and children stay calmer in the midst of disagreements or frustration, thereby enhancing the capacity for rational thought (in both child and adult).
2. Second, Basket B helps child and adult reach mutually satisfactory resolutions to whatever problems or issues (e.g., homework, bedtime, brushing teeth, chores, and so forth) are precipitating difficult interactions in the first place.
3. Third, Basket B teaches a child crucial skills-problem solving, frustration tolerance, delay of gratification, impulse control, and working toward mutually satisfactory solutions-that will serve the child well even in interactions with adults who remain fond of Basket A.

Applying the CPS Approach

Research has shown the Collaborative Problem Solving approach to be highly effective in reducing oppositional behaviour and improving parent-child relations (Greene, Ablon, Monuteaux, et al., 2003). It has also been shown to significantly reduce the number of physical, chemical, and mechanical restraints, locked-door seclusion events, and staff and patient injuries in psychiatric inpatient settings (Greene, Ablon, Hassuk, et al., 2003).

As this is a new approach it is not yet widely available though there are now trained clinicians across the country. Pediatricians should be aware of this new strategy and can promote its principles of understanding how a child's cognitive skill deficits contribute to oppositional/explosive behaviours and teaching parents and children to collaborate may be the most effective of parenting skills.

Final Thoughts

As noted above, the ODD diagnosis is, in some circles, an issue of some controversy. It has been argued that ODD is yet another example of mental health professionals "overpathologizing" developmentally normal behaviour. There is no question that a mere diagnosis cannot hope to capture the complexity of the issues contributing to a child's noncompliance and temper outbursts. Nor are there universally accepted criteria for the frequency or intensity of oppositional behaviour required for children at different ages to be rendered "diagnosable."

Fortunately, a child does not need a diagnosis to have a problem; a child merely needs to have a problem to have a problem. Thus, the question is not whether a child is "oppositional enough" to be called ODD but rather whether a parent feels there is a problem and needs help.

Dr. Greene is Associate Professor in the Department of Psychiatry at Harvard Medical School and Director of the Collaborative Problem Solving Institute in the Department of Psychiatry at Massachusetts General Hospital.

Dr. Ablon is Assistant Professor in the Department of Psychiatry at Harvard Medical School and Associate Director of the Collaborative Problem Solving Institute.

Dr. Miller is Assistant Professor in the Department of Pediatrics at Tufts Medical School and Developmental-

Behavioural Pediatrician at The Centre for Children with Special Needs, The Floating Hospital for Children.

Acknowledgement: The Collaborative Problem Solving Approach study mentioned above was funded by the Stanley Research Institute

The Centre for Collaborative Problem Solving website contains more information on training and lists clinicians trained in this approach.

Underachieving Gifted Students

Underachievement can be simply defined as academic performance that is significantly lower than predicted, based on some reliable evidence of learning potential. It is reasonable to assume there exists a range of mild to severe underachievement. When the discrepancy appears to be significant to the teacher and/or parents, attention should be given to the student's specific needs for modification of educational programming.

WHAT DOES IT MEAN FOR AN INTELLECTUALLY GIFTED STUDENT TO BE AN UNDERACHIEVER?

The concept of an underachieving gifted student may seem inherently contradictory if intellectually gifted students are seen only as those who excel in school at high levels of academic achievement. However, since the new federal definition was formulated in the early 1970s, there has been growing support in the field for defining intellectual giftedness as exceptional potential for high academic achievement, whether or not it has been demonstrated at school. It is assumed that the gifted underachiever has exceptional potential. A student may be gifted in one or many areas of learning or cognitive processing; however, few mentally gifted students have the capability of truly excelling in all subjects and on all kinds of academic tasks.

Gifted underachievers manifest three patterns of Behavioural responses to the school setting: (a) non-communicative and withdrawn, (b) passively complying to "get by," and (c) aggressive/disruptive "problem" students. Behaviour patterns of all three groups tend to reflect feelings of low self-esteem, a lack of belief in their ability to influence outcomes in school, an unrealistic self-concept, and negative attitudes toward school. Generally, these students tend to be loners who have difficulty making or maintaining friendships.

How are Gifted underachievers Identified?

Increasing numbers of intellectually gifted students who have not been recognized and served as gifted because of relatively low patterns of achievement have been discovered over the last two decades as a result of three significant changes in educational practices. First, there has been an increase in the use of tests and sophisticated assessment procedures. Second, there has been an increase in teacher referrals for special education services because of learning or behavioural problems. Third, there has been an increased effort to recognize and develop the potential abilities of culturally different and minority children. Gifted underachievers are also identified as a result of parental accounts of out-of-school behaviours that show advanced interests and skills.

The most disconcerting group of gifted underachievers are those who are not recognized while in school. Awareness of this group has developed primarily through the identification of adults with superior intellectual abilities whose school records show mediocre or poor academic performance.

Why do we need to Identify Gifted Underachievers?

The first reason is obvious — the loss of potential contributions to society from that individual. The second reason is not so obvious — the underachiever's vulnerability to significant mental health and social problems.

Often the gifted underachiever becomes a disturbing behavioural problem both at home and at school. This problem is a natural consequence of the conflict between the individual's personal psychological needs and the lack of opportunities for appropriate learning provided by the school. The third reason is that early identification permits a better chance for reversing patterns of underachievement.

What are some of the Causes of Underachievement?

— LACK OF MOTIVATION. Many highly gifted and creative children have learning styles that are incompatible with prevailing instructional methods. Furthermore, the level of instruction may be inappropriate for these students and the restrictions on learning in the classroom discourage their full participation.

— VALUES CONFLICT. Students may not want to participate in school because of conflicts between the values of the school or the gifted program and the values held by the individuals and/or the cultures from which they come; for example, female students from cultures in which a college education or a career is not expected may underachieve.

— LACK OF ENVIRONMENTAL NURTURANCE OF INTELLECTUAL POTENTIAL. Low socioeconomic status families often fail to provide exposure that stimulates the development of higher level thinking skills. Enriching experiences such as travel, educational activities, and shared problem solving may be neglected. Such students may be from isolated rural settings, economically disadvantaged urban sites, or specific ethnic or cultural minorities that do not encourage intellectual development.

— DEVELOPMENTAL DELAYS OR CHRONIC POOR HEALTH. These students are characterized by relatively low energy levels or interfering hyperactivity. They may have a mild delay in perceptual motor skill development, or a general immaturity in all areas. Often these students have entered school as the youngest in their class.

— SPECIFIC DISABILITIES. Impairment due to specific learning disabilities, brain damage/cerebral dysfunction or neurological impairment, or lack of normal hearing or visual perception may be the cause of underachievement. Some of these students are in fact dyslexic or neurologically disabled. It is not the disability that produces that underachievement but the lack of appropriate programming. These students frequently are not adequately challenged or encouraged to develop their intellectual abilities because of low expectations and a narrow curriculum.

— SPECIFIC OR GENERAL ACADEMIC SKILL DEFICITS. These students may have difficulty with writing, reading, math, or higher level skills necessary for subject matter mastery and high achievement.

After Identifying Students as Gifted Underachievers, what needs to be done? What Educational Programming is Necessary?

Successful approaches to reversing patterns of underachievement have been based on a view that the problem behaviour has been shaped by forces within the school experience and can be altered. These forces essentially are: (a) the social messages conveyed by the teacher and peers that invite or discourage the student to participate (Purkey, 1984) and (b) the degree to which the curriculum and instruction is appropriate for the learning style and performance level of the student. Successful interventions create positive forces to shape achievement behaviour. Programming for gifted underachievers must address three critical areas: (a) an understanding of self— the nature of and problems related to being gifted; (b) development of constructive ways of coping with the inevitable conflict and frustration created by the significant gap between cognitive ability and performance level; and (c) development of a healthier, more realistic self-concept and higher self-esteem.

Effective programming for reversing patterns of underachievement can occur in self-contained classrooms, in resource rooms that provide supplementary services, or through the development of an individual educational plan that may involve a mentor in the school or community. Regardless of the structure, there are five programming components that need to be addressed:

1. The teacher(s) must accept the fact that the student is intellectually gifted, does not want to underachieve or

fail, has low self-esteem, and needs to develop constructive coping skills and self-understanding. The teacher(s) must be skilled in guidance techniques, accurate in understanding the nature of giftedness, and positive in emotional response to the challenge of working with this type of student.

2. The curriculum must be challenging, personally meaningful, and rewarding to the gifted underachiever. There must be a balance between basic skill development and more advanced exploration through the arts and sciences. Career exploration and the development of personal interests are also critical motivating elements, and all learning experiences should be designed for maximum challenge and success.
3. The instruction must require minimal memorization and drill/practice activity and provide maximal opportunity for inquiry, scientific investigation, and creative production. Self-directed learning activities should be encouraged and the students' self-discipline nurtured. The climate created by the instructional style of the teacher should be one of excitement, anticipation, personal satisfaction, and low pressure.
4. The peer group must include at least a few other gifted students, possibly other underachievers, who may become special friends. The group must be accepting of diversity and individual differences.
5. Special services should be provided as needed for handicapped students, for those in need of remedial instruction, or for group counselling. Supplementary psychological and medical services, including family counselling, may also be needed.

Bibliography

Abercrombie, M.L.J.: *Aims and Techniques of Small Group Teaching*, London: Society for Research in Higher Education, 1970.

Anderson, J. E., Ridley, T.: *Cool School: An Alternative Secondary School Experience*, Toronto, Ontario: Institute for Studies in Education, 1977.

Barrows, H.: *Practice-Based Learning: Problem-Based Learning Applied to Medical Education*, Springfield, IL: Southern Illinois University School of Medicine, 1994.

Bottery, M. : *The Ethics of Educational Management: Personal, Social and Political Perspectives on School Organization*, London, Cassell, 1992.

Boud, D., Feletti, G.: *The Challenge of Problem-based Learning*, London, Kogan, 1991.

Bridges, E., Hallenger, P.: *Problem-based Learning for Educational Administrators*, Oregon, ERIC Clearinghouse on Educational Management, 1992.

Burgess, R. L. & MacDonald: *Evolutionary Perspectives on Human Development,* Thousand Oaks, CA: Sage Publications, 2004.

Ellis, B.J., & Bjorklund, D.F.: *Origins of the Social Mind: Evolutionary Psychology and Child Development*, New York, Guilford Press, 2005.

Fordham, P., Holland, D. and Millican, J. : *Adult Literacy, A Handbook for Development Education*, Oxford, Oxfam, 1995.

Galbraith, M.W. : *Education Through Community Organizations*, San Francisco, Jossey-Bass, 1990.

Giroux, H. : *Critical Theory and Educational Practice*, Geelong, Australia, Deakin University, 1983.

Grace, G. : *School Leadership: Beyond Educational Development*, London, Falmer, 1995.

Jacobs, Gregory S. : *Getting around Brown: Desegregation, Development, and the Columbus Public Schools*, Columbus, Ohio State University Press, 1998.

Kakar, Sudhir : *The Inner World: A Psychoanalytic Study of Childhood and Society in India*, New Delhi, Oxford University Press, 1978.

Lovett, T. : *Adult Education, Community Development and the Working Class*, London, Ward Lock, 1975.

MacDonald, K and R. L. Burgess: *Evolutionary Perspectives on Human Development*, Thousand Oaks, CA: Sage, 2004.

Nuna, S.C. : *Education and Development*, NIEPA, New Delhi, 1987.

Okech, J.G.; Asiachi, A.J. : *Curriculum Development for Schools*, Nairobi, Educational Research Publications, 1992.

Rogers, A. : *Adults Learning for Development*, London, Cassell, 1992.

Simkins, T. : *Non-formal Education and Development*, Manchester, Manchester University, 1977.

Smith, M.K. : *Local Education, Community, Conversation, Action*, Buckingham, Open University Press, 1994.

Steele, T. and Taylor, R. : *Learning Independence, A political outline of Indian Adult Education*, Leicester, National Institute of Adult Continuing Education, 1995.

Stenhouse, L. : *Authority, Education and Emancipation*, London, Heinemann, 1983.

White, P. : *Civic Virtues and Public Schooling: Educating Citizens for a Democratic Society*, New York, Teachers College, 1996.

Wilkerson, L., & Gijselaers, W.H.: *Bringing Problem-Based Learning to Higher Education: Theory and Practice,* San Francisco, Jossey-Bass Publishers, 1996.

Woolfolk Hoy, A., & Hoy, W.K. : *Instructional Leadership: A Learning-centered Guide*, Boston, Allyn & Bacon/Longman, 2003.

Index

□□□